Am I Glowing Yet ?

Am I Glowing Yet?

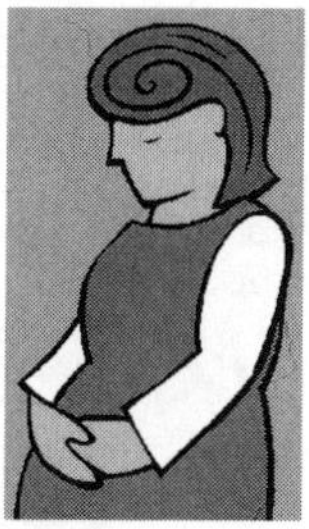

Understanding and Coping with the Common and Not-So-Common Miseries of Pregnancy

Virginia Hege Tobiassen

CHICAGO REVIEW PRESS

Library of Congress Cataloging–in–Publication Data

Tobiassen, Virginia Hege.
Am I glowing yet? : understanding and coping with the common and not-so-common miseries of pregnancy / Virginia Hege Tobiassen. — 1st ed.
p. cm.
Includes bibliographical references and index.
ISBN 1-55652-244-4
1. Pregnancy. 2. Pregnancy—Complications—Popular works.
I. Title.
RG525. T62 1995
618.2'4—dc20 95-36865
CIP

First edition
Published by Chicago Review Press, Incorporated
814 North Franklin Street
Chicago, Illinois 60610
ISBN 1–55652–244–4

5 4 3 2 1

To Kim Ware Malone
and her loving family

Contents

Foreword

Not only is there a paucity of information regarding the topic of this book, which is what I refer to as the "miseries of pregnancy," but little is to be found in professional writings on these matters, especially from the viewpoint of the patient.

Virginia Tobiassen has visited, in a rather complete and comprehensive way, these so-called "not medically serious" occurrences in the pregnant woman's life, bringing to light some of the failures and deficiencies of traditional professional caregiving. Using the specific language of several pregnant women, she not only makes us aware of the true reality of their problems, but provides information to thoroughly and factually discuss each problem and offer the most current research, discussion, and recommendations for treatment of that problem.

Every pregnancy is an adventure of the mind, body, and spirit. It is a unique adventure for the creation of new life, but not without significant challenges. This book will help the pregnant woman meet many of those challenges in a more positive, meaningful way.

William T. Trathen, M.D.

Acknowledgments

WRITING A BOOK IS A LOT LIKE BEING pregnant: It takes a lot longer than you want it to, it makes a hash of your previous life, and it would be impossible to get through without the support of others. I am grateful to everyone who has helped me gestate and deliver this book:

To my clever nephews, Dale and Johnathon Hege, who outgrew their personal computer, and to their parents, Rick and Kathy Hege, who donated the outgrown model to me.

To Rick Palmer, who completed my free-of-charge computer ensemble with the gift of a spare printer he had lying around.

To my parents, Fred and Dolly Hege, who conveniently moved within walking distance of a major medical library and then babysat my son while I did my research there.

To the people whose financial contributions support the Coy Carpenter Library at the Bowman Gray School of Medicine, making it possible for the public to use this fine facility; and to the staff of the library for their unstinting assistance.

To the women who shared their stories for this book: Jan, Linda Sue, Dawn M., Lynette, Betty W., Susan, Mary, India, Patricia, Barbara, April, Kate, Debra Jean, Pam, Bonnie, Carol, Colleen, Linda M., Kim S., Dawn T., Diane, Ann, Linda B., Jae, Kim D., Ramsey, Anna, Louise, Lisa, Dana, Sally, Welmoed, Christy, B.J., Sarah, and Shannon.

And finally, to my husband, Bill Tobiassen, who has supported the family on his remarkable shoulders for the duration of this project; and to our son, Thor Hege Tobiassen, whose gestation unfortunately inspired this book, but who has amply compensated for that beginning ever since the first day he was unleashed on the world.

Introduction

What has happened to your body—the familiar housing you've known all these years? Like the tornado that whirled Dorothy's house off to Oz, pregnancy has snatched your comfortable dwelling off its foundations and dropped it down in a very strange country, with the furniture decidedly rearranged. Maybe you can't remember the last time you kept food down. Maybe you have paralyzing migraines with auras that you think might blind you. Maybe you are bedridden with backache or fatigue, or your skin has broken out in a disfiguring rash, or the palms of your hands itch so badly that you may have to start wearing gloves to keep yourself from gnawing the skin off.

You are suffering a pregnancy that your doctor calls "uncomplicated." But then, your doctor doesn't have to live your life.

The fact is that until you experience it firsthand, it's hard to comprehend just what a miserable pregnancy can do to a life. I know. I used to scoff at pregnancy horror stories. One night at a party I attended during my naively prepregnant years, I overheard my friend Teresa say, "I'd like another child, but I don't think I could stand to be pregnant again."

Come on, I thought. *How bad can it be?*

As proof that there is justice in our universe, a few years later I was served up a miserable pregnancy of my own. Vomiting became the part of my day I most looked forward to. (Happily, I was able to look forward to it several times a day.) Sometimes when I tried to eat, my whole body would begin to shake as soon as the food touched my tongue. Other times I managed to eat, only to feel the top of my head detach itself and float gently to the ceiling after the first swallow. I felt electrically overcharged, as though my body were a pinball machine gone wild, with tiny missiles zooming over my nerves and crashing into each other. Outrageous as it may sound, I will never forget the feeling I had one day that my soul was trying to break out of my body—like a bird beating its wings against its cage—because my body was so sick and my soul so well.

That was how bad it could be—and worse. What made it worse was the message I perceived—from acquaintances, from doctors, from pregnancy books—that if I would just improve my attitude, I could be enjoying my healthy pregnancy.

Because, compared to Teresa's, it really was healthy. Teresa went into preterm labor at twenty-six weeks and was confined to her bed for the next twelve. For all my misery, I remained ambulatory—even on days when that only meant ambling out to the porch to throw up again—and the pregnancy was never threatened. Still, like Teresa, I experienced pregnancy as a complete upheaval of my former life and certainly nothing to glow about.

Unfortunately, I discovered that there is very little support or information available for women suffering miserable but uncomplicated pregnancies. Perhaps this is not surprising, considering that most of the common, nonthreatening pregnancy problems are downplayed in the medical literature as "discomforts" (presumably by persons who have not experienced them). It can be harder to get support while suffering a "discomfort" than while hospitalized with a complication. In fact, far from being regarded as cause for concern, the best-known symptoms of pregnancy are often the source of a lot of good-natured joshing at baby showers. The happy event at the end of pregnancy has a way of casting its miserable symptoms in a rosy light—at least for those not going through them at the time.

Other factors increase the difficulty of finding support. First, despite the number of possible problems, percentages still favor the untroubled pregnancy. For example, while perhaps 70 percent of pregnancies bring nausea in the first twelve weeks, vomiting occurs in fewer than 50 percent, and vomiting severe enough to require hospitalization is probably limited to about 2 percent of all pregnancies. About 16 to 18 percent of pregnant women may suffer severe depression. Disabling back pain may occur in 10 to 30 percent of pregnancies. Estimates for oddball ailments such as unusual skin conditions are sometimes not even available due to lack of study subjects. So for a woman with a miserable pregnancy symptom, the chance of running across someone who can really relate to her problem is smaller than one might expect.

Sadly, cultural and political movements that have improved the lives of women in many ways may have also deprived pregnant women of a supportive environment. For example, when the women's equality movement began to wage war against the notion that biology limited women's roles to home and family matters, it became very important to demonstrate that the functions of women's bodies did not limit their abilities in the workplace. Anything that a male boss might regard as "female troubles" had to be denied, and in fact the movement advanced the idea that only women who *believed* in menstrual or pregnancy problems actually suffered them. It was said that women with meaningful employment would not suffer these problems, because they would have something to think about besides themselves. Betty Friedan foisted this notion on American women in 1963 in *The Feminine Mystique*, claiming that women least afflicted with pregnancy problems "had 'well-integrated egos,' had resources of the intellect and were directed outward in their interests . . . rather than preoccupied with themselves and their sufferings."

As this idea took hold, the women who were babies when *The Feminine Mystique* was published grew up expecting that enlightenment would spare them from suffering in pregnancy. After all, today's M. B. A. s and Ph. D. s can hardly be accused of lacking "resources of the intellect," and most women now confidently expect to pursue their demanding careers throughout pregnancy.

Despite these expectations, some women still find pregnancy a debilitating or incapacitating experience. And despite the changes in women's lives since *The Feminine Mystique*, the percentages of women suffering these problems are about the same as in 1963—with the added complication that today the problems tend to catch women by surprise and with no support system in place for their "female troubles."

Another movement that has backfired in the faces of some pregnant women is the move toward natural childbirth, which has (in some cases quite rightly) taken the medical community to task for regarding pregnancy as something to be aggressively managed rather than a normal process that manages itself. Somehow, in our eagerness to treat pregnancy as a natural state, we have lost sight of the fact that it is also natural to be very sick, to be exhausted, to have pregnancy go awry in any number of ways (some of which resulted in maternal or fetal death before medical doctors interested themselves in pregnancy).

If you believe the myriad pregnancy books currently on the shelf, the natural way to be pregnant is to watch your salt consumption, cut out the caffeine, and then prepare to glow your way through thirty-eight to forty exciting weeks (during which you perform exceptionally well in your demanding job and return home at night to scrub walls, prepare and freeze gourmet meals for after the birth, and blow off your "nesting energy" in a dozen other ways). The relentlessly cheerful tone of most pregnancy books, with their sidebars of can't-fail suggestions for afflictions like "morning sickness" ("Eat a soda cracker before you get up in the morning!") can make the miserably pregnant woman feel worse, as most of these books seem to suggest that pregnancy difficulties can be relieved by living the right life. The corollary suggestion is that a woman with difficulties must be bringing them on herself . . . or imagining them, as the Betty Friedan group holds.

The pregnant woman who takes in these suggestions feels worse because she blames herself. Sadly, many times her friends who have had good pregnancies have also absorbed these ideas (and congratulated themselves for doing everything right), and from these friends the suffering woman may receive subliminal messages of disapproval for her "weakness." As Jan, a three-time sufferer of nausea and vomiting put it, "I think people probably think I'm just not a very strong person and just 'give in' too easily." Perhaps Jan actually received these messages from others through their actions or tone of voice; perhaps she projected her own self-doubts onto others. In either case, clearly she felt a sense of weakness and inadequacy because her pregnancy involved difficulties whose existence is now often downplayed or denied outright. Where such denial is the rule, it can be very difficult for a pregnant woman to find a sympathetic ear, and the resulting feelings of loneliness can make her miseries even harder to bear.

For women who work, pregnancy problems can mean the loss of another important source of support. Contact with friendly coworkers is a morale booster for most people, but a woman sick with a pregnancy may be removed from that circle of acquaintances. She may miss many days because of nausea and vomiting, migraines, or other problems. Even if she makes it to work most days, she may lose her self-esteem or her sense of status in the workplace if she feels that her job performance suffers because of her pregnancy symptoms. Her sense of isolation and her feelings of inadequacy for not being "strong enough" contribute to her unhappiness.

If a woman's normal sources of support are lacking, can she turn to the medical community for help? Unfortunately, women often find their practitioners severely limited in the help they can offer for pregnancy problems. The causes of most miserable pregnancy symptoms are largely unknown, and the only real cure is the end of the pregnancy. Women with "discomforts" such as severe nausea and vomiting, fatigue, headache, backache, or heartburn report very little satisfaction with current treatments. As for a sympathetic ear, some women complain that a physician's experience can get in the way of his compassion for the individual patient. A physician's wife who suffered from nausea, vomiting, and depression in her two pregnancies told me that her husband was sometimes "too clinical" about her problems, that "at some levels he has become desensitized to physical complaints [as well as] to the wonder and mystery of pregnancy." Several other women said simply that their physicians were "uninterested" and seemed impatient with their concerns. Considering the lack of effective therapies for pregnancy complaints, sympathy is often the best an OB can offer–yet sympathy often seems the thing most withheld.

Finally, there are no support groups especially for pregnant mothers, because the special qualities of pregnancy make it a different experience from the kinds that normally inspire such groups to form. First, it is not a chronic disease. No matter how awful things get, every pregnant woman knows the approximate date of her cure. Second, because a happy ending is anticipated, people usually assume that looking to the future is enough to sustain a woman through a difficult pregnancy—even though she herself may be able to look no further than the difficult task of swallowing her supper. And third, when pregnancies end, the former sufferers are usually just too busy to start support groups.

This lack of accessible information, reassurance, or helping hands is not only distressing to a woman in a miserable pregnancy but a departure from the traditions that sustained mothers in earlier times. When our great-grandmothers were giving birth, they could draw on a store of knowledge passed down through many generations; and where knowledge failed, a tradition of heartfelt sympathy and willing hands filled in. Today those support systems have dwindled as great distances separate extended families and women feel pressured to prove their mettle by succeeding in every endeavor on their own.

It is my hope that this book will represent some renewal of those traditions and ties, through the shared stories of other women. Although the book is not an academic study or a work of medical research, it also offers extensive information from the medical literature—though only to acquaint readers with current theories and practices, not to arrive at scientific conclusions. Further, the medical information concerns only pregnancy, as the purpose of this book is not to prepare the reader for labor and delivery—subjects amply covered elsewhere—but to enable her to cope with and understand the problems that may come before.

The women who shared their stories for this book, either through written responses or in personal conversations, do not represent a scientific sample, and no statistics have been calculated based on their responses. What these women have provided is some part of the lost support system—a sharing of knowledge and experience that I hope will bring richness and reassurance to the reader's life.

Taken together, the stories and information that make up this book contain the seeds of five principles that I hope every reader will take to heart:

1. ***You are not alone.*** Even if no one quoted in this book has suffered your particular problem, rest assured that every woman sharing her story (and this group is only a tiny fraction of those with similar tales to tell) understands something of what you are going through. The experience of being miserable when you had planned on being joyful touches most women in similar ways regardless of the particulars.

2. ***It is not your fault.*** Remember, the medical community is still pretty much at a loss when it comes to explaining most pregnancy miseries. This lack of knowledge has not stopped doctors and pregnancy books from espousing timeworn "solutions," and because a sense of authority surrounds these chestnuts, if you find them unhelpful you may wonder what you're doing wrong. Yet you would be hard-pressed to come up with current medical literature that blames you as much as you may blame yourself. Rarely in my research did I come across any evidence that women could avoid the common pregnancy symptoms by changing their habits. Instead, I found the most common feature of these complaints was the etiology (cause): "unknown."

3. ***It is not all in your head.*** Though my mother was having babies in the pre–*Feminine Mystique* era, she did not come to pregnancy with the expectation of being sick. In fact, she knew so little about pregnancy that when she began to suffer intractable vomiting a few months after her wedding, she had no idea what was wrong with her. Hers is an example of how women can be sick without expecting to—and in fact these days it is usually despite their expectations, since many of today's gestating mothers have read all the right books and believe they know how to prevent pregnancy problems.

Further, the fact that your pregnancy has laid you low does not make you weak in any sense. Your sister or coworker or friend did not sail so effortlessly through her pregnancy because she is stronger than you; she simply had better luck. Take pride in the strength that you are displaying by your willingness to suffer pain, depression, or sickness, and to have the rhythm of your life so utterly disrupted, in order to achieve your goal of bringing new life into the world.

4. ***You may need to seek out new options in health care.***

Pregnancy is the only time when the health care choices you make for yourself can directly affect the body of another human. Consequently, you will likely pay more attention to those choices than you ever have before—and you may be surprised at the range of choices available.

A number of women interviewed for this book stressed the importance of finding the right health care provider. "The best thing one can do," said Linda Sue, "is find a practitioner who is sympathetic and to whom one can vent." Dawn M. urged, "Don't take the first OB that comes along. Take the time to choose a caring doctor." She offered this advice to warn others away from her experience, of which she says, "Honestly, I felt like just another cow in the herd. I was down to 99½ pounds from dehydration, and when I did gain some weight back I was 'scolded,' or felt as if I was. I don't remember him being too awfully patient with me—just head 'em up and move 'em out!"

Unfortunately, women in many parts of the country have very little choice in health care providers. If you cannot find the ideal doctor or midwife, make the most of what is available. "You are a consumer of health care," wrote Lynette. "If you feel you aren't getting enough support or the best care . . . at least voice your opinions. Be educated and demand a health care provider take you seriously. These symptoms are *real* and deserve real attention."

Louise, who suffered complications because of problems that were not diagnosed until they had gotten out of control, wrote, "Get a second–or third–opinion! Keep seeking ideas and answers. Seek out possible non-traditional remedies, which doctors may not be familiar with (therefore they often devalue them–be prepared for that!)"

In the United States, "nontraditional" remedies are those that fall outside the standard medical school curriculum. However, many alternative treatments such as herbal medicine, homeopathy, and acupuncture are deeply rooted in traditions whose beginnings predate much of Western medicine. Their long history alone makes them worth pursuing with an open mind. However, you should not set out on this pursuit unaccompanied.

First, try to find an OB-GYN or midwife who is receptive to your search for alternative solutions. Some M.D.s have seen enough evidence of success with nontraditional remedies that they have chosen to incorporate aspects of alternative medicine into their mainstream practices. Whatever your physician's bent, you will likely be happiest if it approaches a match with your own.

Second, if such a match proves impossible, you can still supplement your regular physician's care with the advice of trained professionals in the alternative community. Chiropractors and kinesiologists, herbalists, homeopathic practitioners, acupuncturists–all have their schools and certifications. Perhaps the best combination is your own open mind and your physician's reasonable caution. Many women find that a blend of traditional and alternative medicine provides the best possible management of pregnancy complaints.

5. *It will be worth it!* Not until two days after the birth of my son did I stop to realize (and rejoice) that the nausea of the last nine months had apparently disappeared after delivery. Holding that baby in my arms was so wonderful that I had never paused to reflect on the state of my stomach. I knew then that I would gladly have gone through the whole awful pregnancy again, had it been required of me, for the reward far outweighed the previous nine months' punishment.

Perhaps women with difficult pregnancies have an advantage over the easy-timers when it comes to motherhood. From women who had easy pregnancies I have heard remarks like, "It was all so much easier when the baby was on the inside." It's hard to imagine anyone with a miserable pregnancy ever saying such a thing. There seems to be universal agreement among this group that being a mother beats being a pregnant woman hands down. Whatever the demands of an infant, no human being who has emerged from the womb is likely to cause his mother to vomit every day for weeks on end. The challenges of mothering are infinitely more exciting than the problems of pregnancy, and–hooray!–there are many more support systems, formal and informal, to bear you up in difficult times. But your greatest source of strength will be the love that your baby will bring to your life.

You will not forget the problems of your pregnancy, but they will fade into their proper place in your history as your baby, rather than your body, becomes the centerpiece around which all other life is rearranged. Listen to the voices of the women who have been there, and believe. *It will be worth it.*

1

Nausea and Vomiting

BRACE YOURSELF. HERE IT COMES AGAIN: the smile, the pat on the hand, and the dreaded advice. *Just eat a soda cracker in the morning, and you'll be fine! That's what worked for me!*

Raise your hand if you have fantasized about throwing up on the next person who says this to you. Raise your hand again if you've had this fantasy for six months, or seven, or nine—that is, past the time when everyone assured you your nausea would magically disappear. And one more show of hands, please, if you have been told, or have read, or have felt in your heart that the problem is your attitude.

The problem is not your attitude. The problem is that you are sick. You can't get anything done because every time you stand up, the room spins. You can't eat all those healthy foods the pregnancy books insist on because you gag every time you put food—any food—in your mouth. People ask if you have "morning sickness" and you respond, "Do you mean the 3:00 A.M. vomiting or the 10:00 A.M.?"

Oh, there is an attitude problem—on the part of those who think that the nausea and vomiting of pregnancy (NVP) is something anyone can conquer with soda crackers or a little counseling. This attitude has persisted since around the 1940s, when NVP was regarded as largely or even solely the result of psychological problems—the infamous "all in your head" school of thought. This attitude is problematic because at a very difficult time it robs women of support—from the general public, who may perhaps be forgiven for their ignorance, as all significant writing on NVP is still confined to medical journals, and even from the medical community, who should be better informed by now. A study from the University of Tennessee-Memphis notes that patients hospitalized with severe NVP "garner little attention and engender little sympathy from their physicians. . . . The house staff in obstetrics and gynecology traditionally refer to these patients as 'pukers.'"[1]

Ignorance is the source of the problematic attitude, and there are reasons for the ignorance. While quite a bit of research on NVP has been published in the last five years (much of it by women—inspired by experience, perhaps?), it is not usually a big-money or high-profile subject of inquiry. After all, it is not usually life-threatening, and it always resolves on its own. Further, money from pharmaceutical companies is unavailable for research on NVP because no U.S. drug company has the slightest interest in pursuing medications to combat NVP since the withdrawal from the market of Bendectin, the last anti-NVP pharmaceutical, in 1983. The possible links between medications and birth defects are frightening to drug companies in our litigious society, so frightening that no company is likely now to pursue the development of a drug specifically for use during the crucial early weeks of pregnancy.

Fortunately, it seems likely that researchers with an interest in NVP will continue their inquiries, and their motivation appears to be high. Two researchers whose eyes are clearly open to the realities of NVP made the following observation:

> Nausea and vomiting during early pregnancy may adversely affect a woman's ability to perform work-related tasks, her familial and social relations, psychological status, diet, and health status. . . . Thus, the identification of the factors associated with nausea and vomiting has significant theoretical and clinical implications.[2]

The fact that these researchers refer to nausea and vomiting and not *hyperemesis gravidarum* indicates how well they understand the problems posed by NVP. In some pregnancies—estimates range anywhere from 3 in 1,000 to 1 in 100—a care provider makes the decision to admit a woman to the hospital to restore her nutritional balance and gain control of the vomiting. That decision earns the woman a diagnosis of hyperemesis gravidarum (HG), defined as pregnancy-related vomiting severe enough to warrant hospitalization. Until recently, nearly all the research on NVP focused almost exclusively on cases of HG, discounting as normal any lesser degree of sickness. Although there are generally accepted guidelines that point to the need for hospitalization, including evidence of dehydration, significant weight loss (5 percent of prepregnancy weight is a commonly used figure), and certain findings from blood and urine tests showing a greatly disturbed metabolism, the fact is that a doctor's judgment call, the patient's insurance status, or the availability of hospital beds is sometimes all that separates a hyperemetic pregnancy from one afflicted with normal nausea and vomiting. There is room for a lot of suffering between mild nausea and HG, and researchers are finally beginning to acknowledge that NVP is a significant phenomenon even when it does not put a woman into the hospital.

One of the first problems researchers encounter in studying NVP is determining its true incidence. Estimates vary on how many pregnancies are afflicted with these symptoms. Figures for nausea and vomiting hover around 50 percent, while some estimates for nausea alone go as high as 90 percent. Figuring reliable estimates for nausea is especially difficult because what one woman describes as nausea might be another woman's best day. A woman whose stomach troubles are quelled by a soda cracker might report that she experienced nausea and so figure into a high estimate; on the other hand, women who are disabled or hospitalized by NVP may justly wonder why the soda-cracker set even rates a percentage point.

Because many women do suffer only mild nausea, those with more severe NVP often feel that their colleagues and friends suspect them of hypochondria. After all, their eyes seem to say, how bad can it really be—especially when you get a baby out of it?

The answer is it can be very bad indeed, bad enough that women used to die from the worst cases. Before it became possible to administer fluids and nutrition intravenously, women with intractable vomiting sometimes faced a choice between abortion or death by dehydration and starvation. Sadly, by the time the abortion was performed, a woman was often so debilitated that she died anyway. Given that abortion is now both safe and widely available, one can assume that a woman willing to continue a pregnancy in the face of such severe sickness has a strong commitment to bearing that child. This assumption runs contrary to the pronunciations of the awful all-in-your-head group, who have occasionally had the nerve to suggest that women vomit because they are rejecting the baby.

Perhaps because of such theories, citizens of the twentieth century seem to display less respect for the problem of NVP than any of their forebears. From the first written record of NVP (a papyrus from about 2000 B.C.) until the late nineteenth century, physicians energetically postulated causes and experimented with cures. That is not to say that you, the NVP sufferer, would want to time-travel just to get some respect for your condition, since you would then be subject to the treatments of the past. There is little harm in the earliest prescriptions, such as those found in Soranus's *Gynecology* of the early second century A.D.: body rubs, easily digested foods, and "passive exercise by means of movement in a litter and sedan chair." However, by the nineteenth century, treatments for NVP were invasive and often dangerous. Cocaine, opium, or burning agents (including silver nitrate, carbolic acid, and bromide of potash) were often applied to the cervix. Also common was the forced dilation of the cervix, known as Dr. Copeman's Method. Orally, women received whiskey, various herbs, and morphine. Then there was the doctor who in an 1874 *Journal of the North Carolina Medical Society* described how he had cured a woman of hyperemesis gravidarum by anointing her "three times a day with fresh lard, rubbing it on the inside of the thighs, the groins and under the arms. By thus applying about a half pound of lard three times a day, rubbing it carefully and persistently, it left a soft, silky, delightful state of the skin." One wonders about the doctor's motivation here, but luckily the patient survived (mostly on a diet of iced tea with milk), and at least one person in the room seems to have enjoyed the treatment a great deal.

Even through the first half of the twentieth century, many "treatments" reflected either hopeless confusion regarding the causes of hyperemesis (injections of the husband's blood, intravenous drips of honey) or the belief that its sufferers deserved punishment rather than medical support. An appalling example of the latter, from a paper published in 1934, involved the following directives:

> (a) the banning of visitors to the patient for 48 hours, (b) no vomit bowl to be provided in the room, (c) allow the patient to vomit into the bed and instruct the nurse to be in no hurry about changing the sheets, and (d) instruct the nurse in the patient's hearing to give the patient a fresh meal in twenty minutes if she does vomit.[3]

Fortunately, medicine has come a long way in the management of hyperemesis gravidarum. Rarely do nausea and vomiting threaten the life of a pregnant woman today. Yet there is a large group of women whose quality of life is seriously compromised by nausea and vomiting that bears little resemblance to the "morning sickness" whose description is almost a humorous part of pregnancy lore. "Twenty-four-hour-a-day sickness," as one mother referred to it in our interview, can persist throughout the day or night; it is generally unrelieved by the standard curatives handed out by health care professionals; and It can turn your life upside down.

The severity of NVP usually comes as a surprise to women experiencing it for the first time, many of whom are committed to working at their jobs until their due dates. Trying to carry on with one's career can be extremely difficult in the face of persistent nausea and vomiting, which can make it seem impossible just to keep up with everyday chores, let alone to prosecute an important lawsuit or manage a leveraged buyout. Kate, a freelance writer who suffered extreme nausea and vomiting, says that her first four months of pregnancy "passed in a haze of nausea," during which she did no work and from which she eventually emerged to find a pile of seriously overdue bills on her desk. "I had never missed a payment in my life," she says. "But for four months, there was nothing in the world but me and my stomach."

Betty W. wrote:

> The nausea was debilitating. I would go to the Health Unit [of the EPA office where she worked] and take one-hour naps to get myself back together. This is allowed under federal regulations. Unfortunately, the room was noisy, but it was better than sitting in my office.
>
> I think stress at work may have added to the problems of nausea and vomiting. My second pregnancy went much better than the first I believe in part because I worked just three days a week, not five as I did with the first.

Generous work leave and flexible hours can help the NVP sufferer, but because the symptoms may occur several times each day, it's impossible for a woman to stay home every time she feels sick. Many of the women interviewed for this book had to leave their jobs for some amount of time. Others tried to continue their regular schedules but had to rely on special help, including the understanding of those with whom they worked. Teaching seventh grade throughout her pregnancy, Susan said she often left class to vomit and then taught the rest of the period with wet paper towels plastered to her forehead. Mary, teaching at the college level, was lucky enough to have both her pregnancies begin in the summer when her teaching load was reduced; nevertheless, she likewise reported leaving class to throw up, as well as falling asleep with her head on her desk after each class. Travel to and from work was a problem for Mary as she became very prone to motion sickness, so she kept a resealable bag in her car at all times for emergencies.

India, a nurse, reported that in her first pregnancy she was initially working twelve-hour shifts and had to take Phenergan for vomiting: "It was the only way I could work." In her second pregnancy she was working in a pediatric office with a lighter load, but had to quit anyway. "I was out of work more than I was there," she said.

For those who do manage to keep working, standard coping mechanisms include eating, not just frequently, as most doctors advise, but constantly. A bag of bite-sized foods (nuts, chunks of cheese, small crackers) should always be at hand, and many women also rely on ever-present seltzer water or ginger ale. Of course, constantly stuffing food in your face may get you some strange looks in important meetings, but it is probably preferable to throwing up in front of the company president. Patricia, who taught first grade during her first pregnancy, said she had to find lots of excuses to write on the board so that she could turn her back to the class and slip snacks into her mouth without all her students asking for a share. Betty W. found a useful remedy: "I found chewing gum to be one of the most helpful remedies not listed in any resource."

Whatever you do to cope, don't be surprised or disappointed in yourself if you don't feel you're doing your best work. Remember that your nonpregnant coworkers stay home when they experience the symptoms you're having. No one suggests to them that coming to work will take their minds off intestinal flu or food poisoning. The nature of NVP—long-term compared to most vomiting illnesses, and still often regarded as a matter of attitude—puts you in a position of having to exceed what is expected of others.

What could be more difficult than having NVP while working outside the home? How about having it while you care for other children? Women who experience nausea and vomiting in their first pregnancies are highly likely to repeat the experience. The first pregnancy often seems easy by comparison. Mothers who enjoy giving lots of time and energy to their first children sometimes feel cheated and resentful when sickness from a new pregnancy separates them from their children. Betty W. wrote, "It was tough to spend time with my older child [one year old when the pregnancy began]. I would lie on the couch and do my mothering from there as much as I could." Wrote Barbara, mother of a two-and-a-half-year-old, during her second pregnancy, "I haven't felt energetic enough to engage with my daughter, and I know she senses that. I have felt helpless and a little guilty for my decreasing interaction."

The feelings of resentment and depression that Barbara experienced are not uncommon for women in this situation. Nor are they surprising, considering that the psychological effect of weeks of vomiting is magnified by the guilt or grief a woman may feel over losing time with her other children. Likewise, the physical problems are often magnified by the physical demands of rearing those others, which often preclude the extra sleep and frequent eating that the mother needs to keep her symptoms under control. All mothers interviewed for this book agreed that having other children made pregnancy sickness more difficult. Jan, suffering NVP for the third time, wrote, "My two-year-old gets very tired of Mommy lying in bed and not getting up and getting him things or playing with him. My nine-month-old cries for Mommy a lot and is a lot more fussy."

On the other hand, children are sometimes capable of offering very special comfort. Mary said that her daughter, then about two and a half, would "bring me a pot, or she'd come in the bathroom and pat me on the back while I was throwing up." Even a little child can help by bringing Mommy crackers or a banana, as Mary described her daughter doing. In my own pregnancy, one of my stepsons, then a taciturn twelve-year-old who rarely showed that anyone's feelings had made an impression on him, nudged me one night as we left a restaurant and silently handed me a few packs of crackers he'd saved from his plate. This kind of sympathy can be heartening for a mother, as can the laughter children inspire when you see life through their eyes. "It's pretty bad," commented Jan wryly, "when your two-year-old pretends to be throwing up in his potty."

While only Mom suffers the physical symptoms, a pregnancy afflicted with significant nausea and vomiting affects every member of the family. Younger children suffer the loss of contact with their mother. Older children are better equipped to get by on their own, but they don't like to hear their mother throwing up all the time. Holiday visits can be uncomfortable, as April described:

> We went to visit my in-laws over Labor Day. I was four months pregnant and not vomiting every day, but I still had to eat all the time to keep from getting that sick. On the first night of our visit, my mother-in-law serves this great dinner. But of course, an hour after eating it, I'm thinking, "Oh boy, I'd better eat again." But I was too embarrassed to go sticking my head in the refrigerator while my mother-in-law was still cleaning up from dinner! So I decided to just go to bed, figuring I'd sleep through the sick feeling. An hour after *that*, I was throwing up in the bathroom next to my in-laws' bedroom. Then I was *really* embarrassed.

Whatever other family members do, a husband's reaction to his wife's NVP will probably have the most impact on how well she handles her illness. Support from one's partner is invaluable, but many men have a hard time comprehending the extent of the sickness, and that lack of understanding can lead to tension. Most couples have at least unspoken expectations of each other's contributions to housework, income-producing work, child rearing, social obligations, and sex. It must be upsetting to a man when his formerly competent wife is suddenly unable to achieve much in any of these fields. Any married person, if pressed, would probably admit that it is at least irritating to find one's spouse lying on the couch for hours while the chores go undone. Imagine how the irritating effect multiplies when this behavior persists for weeks. If the wife is hospitalized for vomiting, this effect may be less pronounced, since hospitalization is a sort of note from the doctor excusing the gestating mother from her usual responsibilities. However, in most cases the wife receives no such acknowledgment that she has the "right" to behave this way. Consequently, she usually feels as much guilt as her husband does irritation. Add to all this the fact that her husband has had to move the coffeemaker to the basement so the nauseated woman won't smell the coffee brewing, and tension is bound to surface.

Mary, who was very sick with both her pregnancies, described the kind of conversation her NVP tended to inspire:

> I can remember lying on the couch one night, and I just felt *so awful* . . . and looking at my husband, and just saying the *worst thing*. I said, "Do you like what you have done to me? How do you like what you've done to me?"

Mary added that her husband was "very patient" with this sort of talk. But even this patient man "got tired of me being sick, going into the bathroom to throw up, not being able to cook." And why shouldn't anyone get tired of NVP? The usual cheery assurances notwithstanding, nausea and vomiting do not always pass by the end of the first trimester, and even if they do, twelve weeks is a very long time to experience such disabling symptoms.

If not irritated, the husband may feel, as Susan described hers, "just helpless." It is hard for a loving person to watch a spouse suffer and be powerless to take the suffering away. That feeling of helplessness can lead to a kind of anger. All in all, if your spouse is normally sympathetic and supportive but seems less so when it comes to your pregnancy sickness, perhaps he is just not aware of how miserable you really feel. Even seeing you vomit twice a day may not give him the real picture. Most women agree that NVP is not like any other sickness they've experienced, including viruses that cause vomiting, and that the nausea is impossible to describe. You might try keeping a brief diary for a few days, noting how you feel and what your sickness causes you to do (or stops you from doing) at different times of the day. You may find that putting it down on paper makes it easier to describe, and it may be easier to give your spouse something to read than to tell him face to face. However, even education doesn't guarantee understanding. Barbara, a physician's wife, wrote:

> I'm not sure the ideal sympathetic spouse exists, but I need my husband to understand and say it is OK that I am tired and depressed. I think the fact that he is a physician and has done obstetrics is almost a hindrance because I think he can be too clinical. At some levels he has become desensitized to physical complaints [as well as] to the wonder and mystery of pregnancy.

The support of a friend or relative who has been through NVP can make life easier for the NVP sufferer. Barbara noted that "the most helpful words from a friend to me were the acknowledgment of how bad she felt, how depressed, and how happy to be through with the pregnancy." A friend like this is especially important when other acquaintances seem uncomfortable or bored with the subject of your illness. Mary remembers that her friends were "quietly supportive" but "didn't like to talk about it." Victims of terminal or chronic illnesses sometimes find that healthy friends fall away, whether because they are uncomfortable talking about illness or because the sufferer's symptoms place constraints on social activities. Many women experience something like this with NVP, facing not only a slowdown of their social lives—depressing enough in itself—but a feeling that their illness evokes disapproval among their acquaintances, as Jan described:

> It is depressing not to be able to go places and function like I'm used to because of nausea and vomiting. I think people think I'm just not a very strong person and just "give in" too easily.

Consider Jan's phrasing: *I think people think. . . .* Of course it is impossible to know what people really think. When you try to read minds, part of what you "read" will be based on facial expressions, turns of phrase, and other subtleties; the rest will come from what you feel about yourself as it is projected onto others. Throughout my interviews with NVP sufferers, I was struck by the universality of the feeling that "I am doing something to bring this on myself," as Barbara expressed it. Considering the lack of readily available information on the causes of NVP and the entrenched nature of the all-in-your-head myth, it is not surprising that women, who usually have a strong tendency toward self-blame to begin with, should suspect themselves of somehow provoking their own illness by the failure to do, eat, or *think* the right thing.

This scenario may be particularly common among women who are used to exerting a great deal of control over their circumstances. Many women today enjoy a firm sense of control over their bodies. Education has given them further control of their destinies, and many approach childbearing well armed with information they believe will give them "good" pregnancies with healthy outcomes. It is a terrible shock, then, when NVP robs them of control.

It is human nature to try to assert control over even the most random events, and the typical NVP sufferer naturally tries most any treatment as long as it seems safe for the fetus, from the standard (eating light, avoiding fatty foods) to the outrageous (one caregiver struck my feet with rattles at strategic points). However, most of the women who shared their experiences for this book reported only limited success with any remedy.

Nor is this record of failure surprising. After all, truly successful remedies usually involve some understanding of the ailments they address, and to this day NVP is very poorly understood. However, researchers are currently pursuing a number of different theories focusing on various parts of the body as sources of NVP. Nearly every avenue of inquiry seems to lead at least to possible answers, suggesting that there may never be one narrow answer to why you feel so terrible. With at least six theories out there involving physical causes, plus the die-hard psychosomatic group still coming up with an occasional hypothesis, and every theory seeming at least partially supportable, researchers may eventually agree that NVP is the result of many different bodily disruptions, the combination of which affects every woman in a different way.

With so much research going on, it is surprising and disheartening to find that obstetrical training still includes little information about NVP. A New Jersey midwife notes that she rarely found more than one paragraph on nausea and vomiting in any of the large obstetrical texts she read in her training.[4] Further, any training or discussion regarding NVP usually focuses on hyperemesis gravidarum, leaving the sufferers of "normal" NVP to fend for themselves. Nevertheless, the OB who keeps up with the medical journals will find a good deal of recent research on NVP, most of it centering on the following culprits.

Hormones

Those persons sympathetic enough to reject the all-in-your-head school will usually tell you (with a wise nod) that hormones are responsible for your sickness. However vague this pronouncement, it is one that most NVP sufferers can readily agree with, as it seems the most obvious. Anyone with the most rudimentary knowledge of human reproduction knows that women experience enormous hormonal changes in pregnancy. And in fact, most of the more specific theories about NVP involve the influence of hormones on some part of the body. A basic understanding of some of the hormones associated with pregnancy will help to understand these theories.

The primary hormones influencing pregnancy are the estrogens, progesterone, and human chorionic gonadotropin (HCG). In a nonpregnant woman, the estrogens (comprised of a group of similar compounds, hence *estrogens* rather than *estrogen*) and progesterone are produced by the ovaries and regulate the menstrual cycle. In pregnancy, these hormones are also produced by the placenta, which in addition to its nutritive role for the fetus is also a major endocrine gland. It secretes a special type of estrogen called *estriol*, seen in significant amounts only during pregnancy. It also secretes HCG, which is the hormone that produces the color change on a pregnancy test. Production of HCG begins very early following the implantation of the egg, builds during the first trimester to peak in the third month, and continues throughout pregnancy. The hormone HCG is the key to maintaining pregnancy because its presence signals the ovaries to continue production of progesterone until the placenta takes over that job. Progesterone maintains the uterine lining to support the pregnancy. In a nonpregnant woman, ovarian production of progesterone drops off about fourteen days after ovulation, causing shedding of the uterine lining (menstruation).

Because the hormonal environment of pregnancy is so different from that of nonpregnancy, attention has naturally focused on how elevated levels of hormones might affect parts of the body not immediately concerned with reproduction to produce pregnancy symptoms like NVP. Currently, most attention is centered on the thyroid gland, the liver, and the stomach.

The thyroid. The thyroid gland is a part of the system of endocrine glands. It is made up of small sacs filled with a substance that is secreted by the thyroid to regulate body metabolism and growth. This substance is made up of a protein (thyroglobulin) and the thyroid hormones called *T3* and *T4*. Research has established that pregnant women tend to have elevated levels of these two hormones. In nonpregnant people, these elevations would lead to a diagnosis of *thyrotoxicosis*, a disturbance of thyroid function that is treated with medication. Thyrotoxicosis produces vomiting in some (nonpregnant) patients. In recent years, some researchers have asked whether NVP might be a symptom of a kind of transient thyrotoxicosis produced by the hormonal environment of pregnancy.

Many studies suggest a link between thyroid hormone levels and the human growth hormone HCG, which has been shown to have thyroid-stimulating properties. In particular the presence of HCG seems to correlate with excessive production of T4, and elevated levels of T4 are in turn linked with hyperemesis, showing up in as many as 73 percent of pregnant hyperemetic subjects. But whether HCG is entirely or even largely responsible for the thyroid disturbances of pregnancy remains in question. Even the studies demonstrating a link between HCG and excessive T4 usually find their subjects' concentrations of HCG within a normal range—that is, the nauseated women with high T4 did not show abnormally high levels compared to nonnauseated subjects. Undaunted, some researchers postulate the existence of a variant form of HCG whose stimulating properties work overtime.[5] Such variants have been found in cases of certain cancers in which thyrotoxicosis sometimes occurs as a complication.

Some patients hospitalized for hyperemesis gravidarum have been found actually to have thyroid disease, perhaps preexisting and first becoming apparent in pregnancy. Where other indicators of thyroid problems (such as rapid heartbeat and thyroid enlargement) are present, patients are usually diagnosed and successfully treated for thyroid disease. In other cases it can be hard to distinguish the transient thyroid abnormalities of pregnancy from chronic thyroid malfunction. Doctors warn against rushing into treatment with antithyroid drugs in hyperemetic pregnancies as their use may not be justified. In most cases, thyroid abnormalities tend to resolve themselves as pregnancy continues.

Elevated T4 may be a significant finding in one other aspect of pregnancy. A study of T4 levels in relation to birth weights found that while an excess of T4 did not appear to contribute to intrauterine growth retardation, there did seem to be a correlation between elevated T4 persisting into the second trimester and early labor (before 38 weeks).[6] This study used a very small sample, and no delivery was alarmingly early (the earliest was 36 weeks). However, the researchers suggest that monitoring T4 levels into the second trimester might alert OBs to the possibility of early labor in some patients.

The liver. You may remember from some primeval biology class that the liver is Detoxification Central for the body. Blood passes in and out of the liver at a remarkable rate, about three pints per minute. Cells in the liver help the blood to take in and use the nutrients you ingest and to excrete wastes and toxins. The metabolism of steroid hormones is also under the liver's control, a fact that has recently led some researchers to suggest links between pregnancy hormones, liver function, and NVP.

The liver is an important player in the body's metabolism, including the metabolism of fats, and various conditions of the body can affect the liver by causing excess deposits of fat within it. Among these conditions are diabetes, pituitary disorders, and—you guessed it—pregnancy. A temporary excess of fat in the liver is a normal feature of pregnancy.

Among the fatty substances metabolized by the liver are the *lipids* and *lipoproteins.* In any sort of liver dysfunction, including the changes caused by pregnancy, abnormalities in these substances are common. Many studies have demonstrated an excess of lipids in pregnancy, but one study group found clear and statistically significant differences between NVP sufferers and nonsufferers regarding the composition of those lipids. Since lipid metabolism is influenced by hormones, this finding supports the idea that hormonal influence on the liver can produce changes that lead to nausea and vomiting in pregnancy.

Bile is a product of the liver that plays an important role in digestion (by stimulating the muscle action of other digestive organs and by promoting absorption of nutrients). It also helps to clear the blood of the waste products of red blood cells as they break down over time to be replaced by new ones. From the liver, bile flows into the gallbladder, which stores and releases the substance as necessary. Sometimes an obstruction in the liver or gallbladder can prevent bile from flowing as it should. The condition resulting from stagnation of bile in the liver is called *cholestasis*; in the gallbladder, *cholecystitis.*

Although a diagnosis of cholestasis caused by pregnancy is not very common (estimates range from .02 to 10 percent of pregnancies), it is possible that the conditions leading to such a diagnosis are present to some degree in a much larger number of pregnancies. The symptom that drives pregnant women to their doctors–severe itching, usually in the arms, legs, hands, and feet–generally does not appear until the third trimester. One study of fifty-seven women with this symptom, all diagnosed with cholestasis of pregnancy, found that a high percentage of the subjects had suffered vomiting in early pregnancy and that the vomiting had lasted longer than in women without cholestasis.[7] This finding suggests a link between liver problems and NVP. Similarly, there are strong associations with gallbladder disease and NVP. One study found that every subject who had had confirmed gallbladder disease had suffered nausea in at least one pregnancy.[8] The implication, again, is that dysfunction in this area predisposes a woman to nausea and vomiting in pregnancy, and therefore there is a reason to suspect that the liver plays at least some role in NVP.

If liver problems can cause nausea and vomiting, what is it about pregnancy that causes liver problems? Remember that the liver plays a key role in metabolizing hormones, and consider the rapid increase of sex steroids during early pregnancy. The liver suddenly has a hormone overload to take care of, and some women's livers may simply be less adept at rising to the occasion.

A number of interesting findings support this theory. Perhaps the strongest is a demonstrated association between intolerance of oral contraceptives and NVP. Women who experience nausea and vomiting from the use of birth control pills have a very high frequency of nausea and vomiting when they become pregnant. Researchers point out that just as NVP is most often associated with the first trimester and tends to lessen thereafter, nausea and vomiting with oral contraceptive use often passes after a couple of months. The suggestion is that in both cases the liver eventually adapts to the steroidal load and that it is the initial, rapid increase of hormones that produces the sickness. Early pregnancy produces a higher level of hormonal activity than taking birth control pills, but because pills are taken orally, their steroids move rapidly to the liver from the intestine, and so the total load of steroids on the liver could be similar. One study found that NVP tended to last longer in first pregnancies and to gradually decline if a woman had subsequent pregnancies. The authors of this study postulate that the body eventually adapts to the hormonal changes, comparing it to the way alcohol or drug addiction affects the body.[9] (That is, someone who drinks often and to excess gradually requires more alcohol to experience an effect of drunkenness.) This is an interesting theory, but the women interviewed for this book who had had more than one child did not fit this pattern, though I'm sure they would have liked to.

The stomach. Progesterone, the hormone responsible for maintaining the uterine lining in pregnancy, causes a decrease in the contracting action of smooth muscle tissue. Presumably this reduces the possibility of premature uterine contractions, but the uterus is not the only part of the body affected by progesterone. Smooth muscle tissue also includes the muscles of the stomach that move your food along its digestive path; thus high levels of progesterone in your system make digestion a slower process. It is standard practice to attribute most of the digestive problems of pregnancy, including nausea and vomiting, to slowed "gastric emptying" time. This reasoning has led to the "small, frequent meals" advice you have heard so often. However, studies have not shown that women with and without NVP have any differences in their levels of progesterone. Further, the effect of pregnancy hormones on gastric activity has mostly been studied in animals, because many of the tests involve procedures that present a risk to the developing fetus. These animal data may not present an accurate picture of human digestion.

Whether slowed gastric emptying is even responsible for nausea and vomiting is questionable, since presumably all pregnant women experience this slowdown, but not all are nauseated. One study showed no significant difference in gastric emptying time between pregnant women with and without NVP and concluded that slowed gastric emptying is not responsible for the ailment.[10]

In a letter to the *American Journal of Gastroenterology*, a Dr. M. Mogadam sketched out his thoughts on the causes of hyperemesis gravidarum and described a treatment he claims to have used successfully with a number of patients.[11] According to this doctor, the surge of gestational hormones in early pregnancy causes a reaction in a part of the stomach known as the *gastric pacesetter*, an area that regulates muscular action as food moves from the stomach into the duodenum (the first section of the small intestine through which food passes). The reaction of the pacesetter causes a reversal of this digestive action, so that the contents of the duodenum are forced back into the stomach, producing nausea. Often the contents of the stomach are then forced back into the esophagus, and from there, as any NVP sufferer knows, they are generally forced into the nearest empty vessel.

According to his letter, Dr. Mogadam brought HG to an end with a continuous drip of antacid through a tube placed in the patient's esophagus. He mentions that all the patients undergoing this treatment had tried many antinauseant preparations without success but that the intraesophageal antacid drip brought about quick recovery in all cases, perhaps soothing the irritable gastric pacesetter by reducing stomach acid concentrations.

While Dr. Mogadam's work appears to be unique at this writing—meaning that, unlike many other studies, it has not yet inspired a host of researchers to attempt to reproduce his results—perhaps his new application of a fairly conventional remedy, antacid, will prove helpful to other women in the future.

Dietary Deficiencies

Most people accept the proposition that what they eat is an important factor in how they feel. Many believe that the right foods can prolong life and prevent illness. It is no great leap to imagine that unpleasant pregnancy symptoms such as nausea and vomiting are related to a diet deficient in some important component. This sort of thinking relates to the idea that pregnancy, being a natural condition, cannot itself be responsible for such unbearable illness; therefore (by implication) a woman is responsible for her problem by her failure to keep her body primed with the right foods. These notions are appealing because they lead to the promise that a woman can regain control of her body and her life by controlling her diet. Unfortunately, results of dietary research and experiments have produced little in the way of conclusions or cures.

Probably the most commonly recommended nutritional remedy for NVP is vitamin B_6. At one time it was combined with an antihistamine, doxylamine, to make the prescription drug Bendectin (withdrawn from the market in 1983). However, women interviewed for this book report little success with B_6, either in oral doses or injections. My own experience was dramatically unfavorable. I had received B_6 tablets from a chiropractor who told me that for maximum effect I should chew, not simply swallow, the pills. The next morning at breakfast I bravely crunched into my first dose. The taste was so hideous that my overwhelmed tongue tried to duck down my throat for cover. I will always remember the alarm on my husband's face and the sound of his voice yelling, "Not here! Not here!" as I leapt, retching, from my chair. This experience kept me from trying the pills again, but given the lack of satisfaction other women have noted with B_6, perhaps I didn't miss much.

One study tried loading subjects up with multivitamins before conception to see if dietary fitness could reduce NVP.[12] The subjects reportedly had a lower-than-average incidence of nausea and vomiting when they became pregnant, but of course it's impossible to say how many would have been symptom-free without the vitamins. The researchers in this group note that the multivitamin used in their study did not contain high enough doses of B_6, or any Bs, to link B vitamins to the study findings.

Trace elements such as copper and zinc are coming up for examination in some studies of NVP, with no striking connections so far. There is some evidence that zinc deficiency may be related to pregnancy complications such as preeclampsia, intrauterine growth retardation, and labor problems, but studies have demonstrated that plasma zinc levels in hyperemetic patients are normal and that zinc deficiency probably neither causes nor contributes to hyperemesis gravidarum.

The Corpus Luteum and Its Position

The *corpus luteum* is a fascinating structure that regulates the menstrual cycle in nonpregnant women and helps to maintain pregnancy in the early weeks. In an ovulating woman, one ripened egg is released each month from either the right or the left ovary. The site, or follicle, from which the egg is released actually becomes an endocrine gland that produces progesterone and the estrogens. This gland is the corpus luteum. In a nonpregnant woman, the corpus luteum exists for only about fourteen to sixteen days, then ceases production of hormones and grows over. The body responds to the drop in progesterone by shedding the uterine lining, and the cycle begins again.

In pregnancy, the corpus luteum remains active for a time, continuing to produce its secretions. An ultrasound during pregnancy can determine whether the corpus luteum is on the right or left ovary, a technique used by one group of researchers to study whether the site of the corpus luteum had any effect on nausea and vomiting during pregnancy.[13]

One reason the researchers pursued this possibility was that if it held up to testing, it might explain why some women are sick in one pregnancy and not in another. Anatomy also pointed in this direction, since the veins of the right and left ovaries drain into different structures, and it is possible for hormones draining from the right (but not the left) ovary to be carried directly to the liver via the portal vein. The group putting forth this possibility is one of the original proponents of the theory that hormonal load on the liver is responsible for NVP. From this perspective, it certainly makes sense that corpus luteum hormones draining directly into the liver would cause sickness.

The study did indeed show a strong correlation between right-side corpus luteum and NVP. Of the subjects with nausea and vomiting, 69 percent had a corpus luteum on the right ovary. Of the women who experienced no nausea, 88 percent had a left-side corpus luteum.

A few years later, an interesting case seemed to cast some doubt on the right/left theory.[14] In this case, a woman with severe NVP had her corpus luteum surgically removed at twelve weeks because it had formed a cyst that produced intense abdominal pain. Consistent with the right/left theory, this NVP sufferer had a corpus luteum on the right ovary. However, its removal did not alleviate the nausea and vomiting; in fact, they became more pronounced, and when no therapy proved effective, the patient finally requested an abortion.

The doctors involved in this case argue that if hormones draining from the right-side corpus luteum were responsible for NVP, this woman would have been cured of her symptoms by removal of the corpus luteum. However, with so many other theories in play regarding the cause of NVP, it certainly seems possible that nausea and vomiting in pregnancy could be related to more than one factor, and that the woman in this case may have had other conditions contributing to her symptoms. The right/left theory has been neither proved nor disproved by any large-scale studies. An editorial in *Obstetrical and Gynecological Survey*, while calling the theory "interesting to contemplate," remarks that "it is hard to imagine that nature made this mistake."[15] On the other hand, a woman suffering NVP may not regard this as a great leap of imagination. After all, if Mother Nature thinks that disabling nausea and vomiting is the proper way to herald the beginning of a new human, of what other hideous misjudgments might she be capable?

Psychological Theories

Every nauseated pregnant woman has the right to keep and ponder in her heart the following piece of information:

> There are very few who now think that persistent nausea and vomiting arise from emotional problems in the patient's life or in her relationships with others.
>
> —editorial, *Obstetrical and Gynecological Survey*.[16]

Unfortunately, while that may apply to researchers studying NVP, it does not seem to capture the mindset of the general public or of some OB-GYNs. The belief that NVP is all in the head has been with us for a very long time, and despite the amount of current research going against it, it seems to be as intractable as the vomiting. To give you an idea of what the NVP sufferer is up against, as well as to arm you with a bit of information from behind enemy lines, a little history of this theory may be helpful.

Until the late 1800s, theories about the causes of NVP were centered on physical causes. The first psychological theory receiving wide notice was an 1891 paper by R. Kaltenbach, who stated that "the vomiting of pregnancy is usually a manifestation of neurosis, somewhat allied to hysteria."

Early explanations for the physical causes of NVP have rightly been dismissed as products of their time. (For example, the idea that NVP was caused by "an abundance of humors gathered together in the stomach," put forth in 1609, comes from a time when the idea of bodily humors dominated medical thinking.) Yet Kaltenbach's theory has persisted, its proponents apparently disregarding how the good doctor's era (when neuroses were the height of fashion for women) might have skewed his thinking.

From the 1930s through the 1950s, medical writing took Kaltenbach to greater and greater extremes, resulting in a barrage of withering indictments of the mental fitness of the NVP sufferer:

> Menninger [1943] thought that vomiting in hyperemesis was due to "a repudiation of femininity," while Weiss and English [1943] suggested that it was due to "a conscious or unconscious wish not to become pregnant." . . . In some instances the basis was an unconscious belief that a sin had been committed, and because childhood fantasies suggest that pregnancy had taken place by way of the gastrointestinal tract, the unconscious desire to be rid of the fetus produced an attempt to expel it the same way.[17]

The year 1943 was apparently the high (or low) point of this kind of thinking. That was also the year that M. B. Hall, writing in the *Journal of the American Medical Association*, claimed that animals do not suffer nausea and vomiting during pregnancy because "the female animal is free from any sense of shame in the presence of its mother and does not submit to coitus from a sense of duty to the male, as is suggested to be the case with the human female."[18] Dr. Hall failed to mention that while no other animal but the human sheds tears when it grieves, doing so is not usually regarded as evidence of psychological problems. Nor did he apparently consider that human beings talk, think, write novels, build buildings, and make amazing scientific discoveries, but in most cases not because they are ashamed of themselves in front of their mothers.

While those currently exploring physical causes of NVP naturally question the correctness or completeness of psychological theories, you might expect the members of the psychiatric community to stick together. In fact, they don't. Studies in psychiatric journals tend to have conflicting results leading to contrary opinions. For instance, many of the all-in-your-head school are still operating on the assumption that vomiting indicates that a woman doesn't want to be pregnant. Yet the greater number of studies have failed to support this connection, finding no correlation between NVP and the circumstances surrounding the pregnancy including marital status, planned versus accidental pregnancy, practical hardships such as financial difficulties, or even whether a subject expected to be sick.

My own experience, like that of many women interviewed for this book, clearly demonstrates the lack of correlation between desire, expectations, and NVP. First of all, I was certain I would not be sick, because I knew all the "right" things to do. Further, I eagerly anticipated pregnancy for months after my husband's five-thousand-dollar vasectomy reversal. When it finally happened, I was ecstatic—until a few weeks after the pregnancy test, when I was too sick to move anything but my eyes. Desire to have the child was the thing that sustained me—not the thing that sickened me.

Some papers have pointed out that selection methods for psychological studies of NVP are usually flawed, skewed toward psychiatric patients and not including controls. Further, there is the problem—which only a few, observant authors have noted—that cause and effect are easily confused in dealing with NVP. A woman with severe NVP may well be depressed and anxious, but is she sick because of her depression, or is she depressed because her body is out of her control, her life ravaged by constant nausea and vomiting? One study found that the attitude most strongly correlated with NVP was neither acceptance nor rejection of the pregnancy, but ambivalence. Surely ambivalence is not surprising, even with a much-desired pregnancy, when a woman has been vomiting for weeks. As several papers mentioned, interviews for these studies are usually done during the period when nausea is most severe. At such a time, most women are likely to say something like Christy did: "I thought it was not worth it at the time. I remember telling friends, 'This is supposed to be wonderful, but I am not impressed one bit with pregnancy.'" Undoubtedly, a psychiatrist interviewing Christy would have called this "ambivalence," but Christy was simply tired of being nauseated.

One doctor who treated many women for hyperemesis gravidarum stated that his patients' initial apprehension and depression were caused by their severe sickness, not the causes of that sickness. The patients he dealt with often faced a choice between continued hyperemesis or abortion, a choice likely to depress and overwhelm anybody. This doctor noted that when the patients' nausea and vomiting ceased, their "pseudo-psychiatric disorders" vanished as well.[19]

A good example of how cause and effect might be confused comes from a 1988 study that attempted to relate first-trimester vomiting to items on a scale of stressful circumstances such as the death of a child, injury of a loved one, loss of a job, and unwanted pregnancy.[20] When few of the stressors on the scale showed up in any significant numbers in the 102 study subjects, researchers added three of their own: "poor communication with my husband," "stress, doubts, and inadequate information about pregnancy, childbirth, and health of fetus," and "poor communication with obstetrician." Many women participating in this study agreed that they had experienced these stressors, leading the researchers to speculate that these factors might cause women to vomit as a symbolic rejection of pregnancy.

To understand how such a study could confuse cause and effect, imagine what a typical NVP sufferer might say to a friend: "It's been so hard. I can't seem to make my husband understand how sick I am. I feel scared because none of the pregnancy books say anything about being this sick, which makes me wonder if something's wrong—but my doctor never says anything about it." A researcher eavesdropping on this conversation would no doubt check off all three of the study's added stressors based on this woman's comments. Yet she feels these frustrations and fears as a result of her sickness. If her physical functioning were normal, perhaps none of these problems would ever come up.

Actually, studies like this one aside, the literature of psychiatric medicine is full of good news for NVP sufferers. First, there is the hope that the all-in-your-head school is closing its doors. Most of the recent papers on NVP balance their findings with an acknowledgment of the evidence for physical causes, often saying that mental disturbances may simply exaggerate a physically generated condition.

But the most cheering news is that evidence now argues for NVP as a sign of *healthy* mental functioning. Some studies have shown that women with severe nausea and vomiting in pregnancy tend to adapt better to life with a new baby and have fewer postpartum problems. Women who have suffered NVP would likely offer a simple explanation: Most anything a baby can do on the outside is easier to deal with than the problems it caused on the inside. The new mother may not have much control over her hours, but she has control of her body again. However, those who seek their explanations in the realms of the subconscious propose that complete *absence* of nausea in pregnancy could sometimes result from repressed feelings about or denial of the pregnancy. So let it all out, ladies–you can always mop it up later–and be glad that your psyches are in such good shape, even if your bodies can't get out of bed before noon.

Feeling Better

While doctors have developed successful methods of controlling hyperemesis gravidarum, the in-between patient–meeting the criteria neither for IV therapy, nor for what used to be a life–may try many types of remedies without success. No woman interviewed for this book reported any treatment that brought her digestive system back to normal. Some were able to control their vomiting with prescription anti-emetics, but none found a way to banish the nausea or even to carry on completely with her regular activities.

Since the cause of NVP is still unknown, current medical practice is to offer dietary suggestions and to treat the symptoms (for example, give an anti-emetic to control the vomiting–which does not address the cause but suppresses the symptom) when they become intolerable. The dietary advice centers around light eating at frequent intervals. This advice, which is in the repertoire of every OB caregiver and reproduced in every pregnancy book, is popular because it seems logical and certainly poses no risk to the fetus. It is also, for many sufferers of serious

NVP, almost completely worthless. As for logic, most of the dietary suggestions are based on the assumption that nausea in pregnancy is caused by a disturbance in the action of stomach and intestines, while much of the current research suggests otherwise.

If you are suffering severe nausea and vomiting, you will adjust your eating habits to whatever works for you, and what works will probably be highly individual. Most women in this situation don't need to be told to eat frequently. They will be either compelled by their bodies to do so or unable to eat no matter what anyone says. As for foods to avoid, the woman's body likewise directs her in these choices. A sensible diet for the NVP sufferer's first trimester may be whatever she can swallow without gagging.

Medications. The only drug approved by the FDA specifically as a remedy for NVP was Bendectin, which appeared on the market in the mid-1950s and was withdrawn by its manufacturer in 1983 after a number of lawsuits charged that the drug had caused birth defects. Dawn M., pregnant in 1974, took Bendectin: "It was the only thing that kept me alive. I knew I could not function without it." Today, Dawn said, "I feel the nausea prescription may have affected my daughter in that she always seemed to have trouble in school with concentration—possible learning disabilities—although I never had her tested. Learning disabilities have just been focused upon, and my daughter is almost twenty."

No study ever conclusively linked Bendectin to birth defects, but the court battles are still going on. Meanwhile, the two active ingredients of Bendectin are available over the counter. One of them is vitamin B6, or pyridoxine, whose use against NVP dates back at least fifty years (see discussion later in this chapter). The other component was doxylamine, an antihistamine. (Antihistamines have an effect on the central nervous system that suppresses the urge to vomit.) Doxylamine is available in an over-the-counter sleeping aid, Unisom. Some physicians "bootleg" Bendectin by recommending a combination of B6 and Unisom to their patients. However, the Unisom package clearly bears a warning against use of the product in pregnancy. Bear this in mind and discuss it thoroughly with your doctor if he or she suggests this combination to you.

Anti-emetic (antivomiting) drugs do exist. Some of them are used in pregnancy, though none is specifically formulated for pregnant women, and studies have suggested that some may pose a risk to a developing fetus. A nonprescription type of anti-emetic is a combination of sugars and phosphoric acid (the latter to control stomach acidity). Brand names include Emetrol, Especol, and Controflex. These have never been proved effective in combating pregnancy vomiting, but medical writers suggest they are not likely to be of any harm in pregnancy, unless the woman is diabetic (because the preparations are almost all sugar).

Prescription anti-emetics and their brand names include the following[21]:

buclazine (brand name Bucladin–5), cyclozine (brand name Marezine), and meclazine (brand name Antivert): Drugs in this group are usually prescribed for motion sickness. Medications in this group have produced birth defects in rats when given early in gestation.

scopolamine: Once upon a time, this was given to women in labor as an amnesiac–something to make them forget the whole experience in the "twilight sleep" induced by the drug. Today scopolamine is given as an anti-emetic, usually in the form of a skin patch. Despite its having been in use for years, no controlled studies exist on its effects in animal or human pregnancies.

promethazine (brand name Phenergan): This drug has no reported link to birth defects but should not be taken in the third trimester, when it is associated with a risk of increased jaundice in newborns.

chlorpromazine (brand name Thorazine) and proclorperzane (brand name Compazine): No studies indicate that these have an effect on the fetus in the first trimester, but they should not be taken in the third trimester, when they are associated with an increased risk of jaundice in newborns. Possible side effects include muscle spasms, blurred vision, and movement problems.

Of the medications above, Phenergan is probably the drug most commonly prescribed for NVP. Several women interviewed for this book used Phenergan when vomiting threatened to obliterate their working lives. Jan said, "Phenergan didn't make me feel any better; I did hesitate [to use it, for fear of fetal effects] and didn't use it as much as was recommended." Susan resorted to Phenergan "to keep from going into the hospital" in her first trimester but noted that the drug did little more than prevent hospitalization. It controlled her vomiting enough to forestall dehydration but did not relieve her insistent nausea. India took Phenergan in order to continue her demanding twelve-hour shifts as a nurse, but like Jan and Susan, didn't feel much better for it. An anti-emetic like Phenergan is not a wonder drug. In pregnancy it is usually prescribed, as it was for Susan, in an attempt to break the cycle of vomiting and help a woman get control of her nutrition again.

While doctors hand out diet tips and the occasional prescription drug, NVP sufferers are out there trying anything and everything to regain control of their lives. The successes women report are usually small victories, things that help "a little." Also, remedies are often successful only on an individual basis, suggesting again that NVP is a complex ailment that affects every woman differently. So it is that every sufferer must seek out her own coping strategies. Below are some places to begin your search.

Acupressure. In ancient Chinese medical theory, acupuncture (today often replaced by acupressure, less threatening to skeptical Westerners) was believed to restore the balance of positive and negative energies flowing through the body. Specific locations were stimulated depending on the type of ailment. For instance, stimulation of the *nei kuan*, a point on the forearm, was a method of preventing difficulties in early pregnancy, preventing and treating eclampsia, and improving lactation after childbirth.

Current thinking on acupressure and acupuncture is that stimulation of the skin in appropriate places results in the production of endorphins, morphinelike compounds produced by the body that can modulate pain, stimulate the release of some hormones, and positively affect emotion and behavior. Coupling this modern theory with the directives of the ancient methods, some researchers are now looking at stimulation of the nei kuan as a way to relieve nausea and vomiting in pregnancy.

A study tested acupressure wristbands, designed to stimulate the nei kuan, for their effect on both NVP and the emotional state of early pregnancy.[22] This study pointed out the correlation between nausea and vomiting and psychological problems such as anxiety, depression, and hostility—that persistent nausea leads to these psychological problems, and not the other way around. Study subjects showed significant improvements in both physical and mental status after brief use of the acupressure wristbands, and some whose nausea was not relieved still found their emotional state much improved.

Unfortunately, this study used a very small sample, and there were problems that make the data less than completely reliable. However, you can do your own personal study with wristbands, available under the brand name Sea Bands. (One source is the Natural Baby Company, [609] 771-9233.) Or you can try applying pressure to the nei kuan with the fingers of your opposite hand. The point is located on the underside of the arm, a distance of three fingers' width from the wrist crease, between the two tendons there. Another pressure point to try is on your chest. Find the sternal notch, a small depression at the bottom edge of the breastbone. The pressure point is just above that notch. Try pressing it whenever you feel a wave of nausea.

Vitamin B_6. The use of vitamin B_6 as a remedy for nausea and vomiting in pregnancy was first written up in a medical paper in 1942. Many studies since then have proclaimed the effectiveness of B_6. The most recent[23] reported that while oral doses of B_6 (25 milligrams every eight hours) made no difference in mild to moderate nausea, women with severe nausea experienced significant improvement. All subjects with vomiting felt that B_6 reduced the symptom.

Some women report a difference in effectiveness depending on the time of day that they take B_6. Nighttime doses may be more effective than morning doses. Nutrition advocates counsel pregnant women to eat foods rich in B_6 to prevent nausea. These include meats, fish, chicken, eggs, brewer's yeast, and whole grains such as brown rice. However, it is doubtful that foods can provide enough to make a difference. The medical literature suggests at least 50 milligrams a day above dietary sources, but discuss any larger dose with your doctor, as excessive B_6 has been linked to symptoms of nerve damage (see Chapter 3). You can also ask your doctor for B_6 injections, which may work for you if you have a problem swallowing the tablets.

Exercise. If you are capable of moving at all, try moderate exercise. Several women interviewed for this book found it helpful, as Kate describes:

> Even though it was difficult to get moving, I found that slow, careful walking coupled with rhythmic breathing helped me. It didn't take the nausea away, but it felt like it stabilized me, made the boat stop rocking.

Be sure to keep your exertions within reasonable limits. Vigorous exercise may leave you exhausted, dehydrated, and overheated—conditions likely to increase nausea.

The prescription for moderate exercise is in line with the ancient advice of the Greek physician Soranus, who during the second century A.D. recommended "active exercise in the form of dancing, punching the leather bag, playing with a ball." He also recommended exercise of the voice and reading aloud "with modulation," a prescription that is not as farfetched as it may sound. Two women interviewed for this book report that *singing* was one of their most effective weapons against nausea. Debra Jean discovered this technique when her musical group refused to let her sit out a performance despite her intense nausea. By the time she got offstage an hour later, her nausea was much improved, and she used singing to combat sickness for the rest of the pregnancy and again in the next one. She credits the controlled breathing used in singing with dispelling the nausea. Kate also used singing, "especially hymns, the slower the better." If you don't believe you have anything to sing about, breathing exercises or, as Soranus suggested, reading aloud may produce the same calming effect.

Food and drink. Food tolerances and aversions among NVP sufferers tend to be highly individual, and they often defy the conventional wisdom. After weeks of eating nothing, I suddenly found that fast-food burgers and french fries—foods I hadn't eaten in years—settled my stomach in a wonderful way. On the other hand, Susan reports that in her best phase she could tolerate only the conventional bland foods: "cottage cheese, bagels, crackers, mashed potatoes. We joked that I could only eat white things."

A food may work for a while, then suddenly disgust you, as Kate describes:

> Watermelon was my salvation at first. Then suddenly I got grossed out just looking at watermelon. But by then my husband had got-

ten hooked on watermelon, so every time I opened the refrigerator, there it was! It was awful!

Carbonated drinks are often helpful. Seltzer or mineral water helps some women. Ginger ale also works for some, perhaps because of the ginger, which is supposed to have properties that suppress nausea (see discussion of ginger later in this chapter). Coke is also famous for its stomach-settling quality and is available in a caffeine-free version. If one drink makes you retch, try another—you might find the right formula for you.

When I was a child, a severe vomiting virus swept through my school. I was felled for at least a week but recovered uneventfully, while my best friend was hospitalized for dehydration. Possibly I fared better because my mother gave me, every half-hour, a spoonful of a nasty-tasting beverage she had concocted according to the pediatrician's recipe. This weak solution of water, sugar, and salt apparently kept my electrolytes in balance. Research for this book turned up a similar recipe to be used for vomiting in pregnancy:[24]

⅓ cup lemon juice

⅓ cup honey

¼ teaspoon salt

1 calcium tablet, powdered (not bone meal or dolomite)

Water to make one quart

Try taking spoonfuls of this at regular intervals.

A word about eating from Jane Martin of the Natural Baby Company: "Hunger is a feeling of the past. If you don't feel hunger, just translate *nauseous* into *hunger*." This is excellent advice. Don't wait for hunger pangs, because they may never come. Many of your body's familiar responses and signals will be different in the presence of continuous nausea.

Ginger. The use of ginger as a remedy for gastrointestinal problems dates back hundreds of years. One study cites research suggesting that ginger's absorbent properties may reduce stimuli from the stomach to the so-called vomiting center located in the brain stem.[25] Ginger also has carminative properties—that is, it helps expel gas from the intestines and relieves crampy tummyache pain. Subjects in this study took daily 1 gram doses of ginger. Nineteen of twenty-seven subjects reported that nausea and vomiting were diminished through the use of ginger.

There are ginger pills, ginger ale, ginger teas, and other preparations available. Unfortunately, no one interviewed for this book reported much relief from ginger, but it is still worth a try. What isn't?

Herbs. Carminatives such as peppermint, spearmint, and fennel have all been suggested. However, carminatives are believed to exacerbate heartburn (see Chapter 6), so you may be in a can't-win situation with these. Raspberry leaf tea is supposed to be helpful, as is anything with a high tannin content (including regular black tea, which is available decaffeinated in case you are restricting caffeine).

Homeopathy. Homeopathy is an alternative medical practice that is gaining popularity in the United States. Based on what is called the Law of Similars, it treats symptoms with extremely dilute solutions of substances that in full strength would produce similar symptoms. For NVP, for example, a homeopathic practitioner might administer a dose of ipecacuanha (or ipecac), because it is a plant that causes vomiting when ingested. Other homeopathic remedies for NVP might include *Colchicum autumnale*, natrium phos, nux vomica, or phosphorus.

Please be aware that homeopathic medicines are made by special pharmacies according to an official, FDA-recognized manual. The original substances are diluted to one part per million. Some of these substances are poisonous at higher strengths. So while correctly prepared homeopathic solutions may be self-administered without risk, *do not* attempt to make your own solutions, and never take the original substance at any dose.

Hypnosis. I admit to a prejudice in favor of this therapy. When I sought out a hypnotherapist in my second month, I had been unable to swallow more than a bite or two of any food for a couple of weeks. When the therapist asked me what suggestion I wanted her to introduce in the trance, I said, "I would like to believe that *food is good.*" I also said a general suggestion of happiness would be nice, since I was so miserable at a time when I wanted to be celebrating.

When I left the therapist's office, I drove straight to the nearest restaurant, opened the menu, and was dazzled by how delicious everything sounded. I ate an omelet and salad, my first real meal in two weeks. The rest of the day I walked around with a goofy grin on my face, occasionally wondering why I felt so happy and then remembering that I had asked the therapist to make me feel that way.

The therapist also taught me a self-hypnosis routine incorporating feelings and goals I had expressed in our interview. At least once a day I spent about twenty minutes in this exercise. It wasn't as powerfully influential as the therapist-induced trance, but it definitely helped me feel more calm and in control of my body.

The fact that hypnosis can assuage nausea or control vomiting does not mean that NVP is all in your head. People undergo dental work and even surgery under hypnosis, and no one would presume to suggest that the pain of being drilled or cut open is produced by a bad attitude. Hypnosis is also used to help chemotherapy patients overcome nausea and vomiting. The mind is a powerful force that, properly focused, can override the physical sensations within the body.

Incidentally, when my obstetrician signed a form stating that I had undergone hypnotherapy for hyperemesis gravidarum, Blue Cross paid for my session. Keep it in mind (no pun intended).

Staying cool. You may find that your nausea is greatly exacerbated when you feel overheated—which you will, especially if your early pregnancy falls in the warmer months. Mary says that staying cool by floating in a swimming pool was helpful in relieving her NVP. Kate says she took walks in the cool, ("around forty-five degrees") early mornings of September and found the coolness soothing. Cool washcloths on the forehead and cold packs on pulse points are traditional chillers that may relieve the worst of your nausea.

Avoidance. Obviously, you will avoid whatever makes you feel ill if you can identify it. But there is one substance strongly associated with nausea that most pregnant women ingest every day: supplemental iron. According to many sources, including the World Health Organization, iron supplementation may not be necessary in most pregnancies and should in any case be delayed until at least the second trimester. If you are in early pregnancy, nauseated, and taking iron tablets, ask your doctor if you can hold off on the tablets until your stomach settles down.

Treatment for Hyperemesis Gravidarum: What to Expect If You Are Hospitalized

Everything about hyperemesis gravidarum—from diagnosis to treatment to decisions about what constitutes recovery—seems to allow a great deal of room for the opinions and practices of individual doctors within a skeletal set of guidelines drawn up half a century ago. Those guidelines, established in 1956 by the American Council on Pharmacy and Chemistry, suggest that a diagnosis of HG apply only to patients "who develop intractable vomiting and disturbed nutrition, such as alteration of electrolyte balance, loss of weight of 5 percent or more, ketosis, and acetonuria, with ultimate neurological disturbances, liver damage, retinal hemorrhage, and renal damage."

Some of these guidelines are unreliable, such as the "5 percent" rule. Not every woman states her prepregnancy weight accurately, so the percentage may be off the mark. You would also hope that your illness would never go far enough to display any of the "ultimate" characteristics of the HG patient. That leaves laboratory findings as the best measurement of the severity of nutritional disturbance. For this reason, your doctor will likely request blood and urine samples just prior to or upon your admission to the hospital. These samples can also help to rule out unexpected causes of vomiting such as thyroid disease or bacterial infections.

Standard hospital treatment of HG includes IV therapy for nutrition and fluids. Eventually you will receive small amounts of fluid by mouth to test your ability to keep things down. The idea is to give the gastrointestinal tract some resting time to break the cycle of vomiting; that's why most patients receive nothing by mouth at first. However, Lynette, who was hospitalized for HG, said:

> During severe hyperemesis, between hydration, they told me to sip fluids and not stress my body with solids. I, however, knew that I had to at least nibble saltines to keep the fluids down. I convinced my husband to bring me saltines and finally kept small amounts of fluids down.

Just because you are in the hospital doesn't mean you have to succumb to what Dawn M. described: "I remember feeling that I was at the mercy of the medical profession to keep me going." Remember that a lot of this therapy is still based on trial and error, educated guesses, and the particular prejudices of individual doctors. If you feel strongly that something isn't working for you, insist that your doctor take you seriously.

As the IVs do their work, your ability to tolerate oral nutrition should improve, and your doctor will attempt to build it up gradually. Some doctors add drug therapy to this routine.

When will you be released from the hospital? The proper time to pronounce an HG patient "recovered" has come up for argument in the literature. The common marker for release is cessation of vomiting, but several studies suggest this measure of wellness is inadequate and leads to repeat hospitalizations. Denys Fairweather, whose 1968 paper "Nausea and Vomiting in Pregnancy" is still the standard work on the subject, feels that the most common cause of repeat admission for HG is releasing the patient too soon the first time. He recommends that the patient show evidence of steady weight gain before release.[26] Then again, he was writing at a time when hospitalization did not so often bankrupt the patient. At any rate, you may wish to discuss this recommendation with your doctor if you feel you are at risk for recurrent hyperemesis gravidarum.

Outcomes

There is a bright side to NVP, and though you may find it of rather distant interest while your head is in the toilet, on some level of your subconscious it may fortify you throughout this difficult time. Women who vomit in pregnancy run a much-reduced risk of early miscarriage (before twenty weeks), compared to women with no nausea or vomiting. You may have heard this as folk wisdom, but statistics bear it out. Some researchers theorize that a woman with no NVP may not be producing sufficient levels of the hormones needed to sustain her pregnancy and thus may be at risk for early spontaneous abortion. So if your physician seems unconcerned about your nausea and vomiting, remember that one of the obstetrician's first duties is to ascertain the health of the pregnancy. He or she may simply have placed an approving mental checkmark next to your symptoms and neglected to consider their effect on your life.

A possible exception to the sick mom–healthy baby equation is the untreated case of hyperemesis gravidarum. Some studies associate hyperemetic pregnancies with low birth weight, fetal growth retardation, central nervous system problems, and skeletal malformations. Though none of these associations is without its detractors, all may play an important part in the decisions facing the hyperemetic woman and her caregiver. Several studies point out that when assessing birth defects in hyperemetic pregnancies, it is sometimes impossible to determine whether defects resulted from drugs taken to control the vomiting or from the mother's hyperemesis. Nutritional deficiencies resulting from intractable vomiting may present more danger to a fetus than drug treatment, particularly since many of the common anti-emetics have so far not demonstrated any association with birth defects. At any rate, if a woman meets the accepted criteria for HG, it is vital that her nutritional balance be restored in some way. Modern medicine's ability to do so is what prevents HG from threatening the mother's life or necessitating an abortion as it did in previous centuries.

Admittedly, those modern practitioners who *protect* your life can't do much to help you *enjoy* it during your bout with NVP. That is a challenge perhaps best left to your inner resources, which at least will never do any harm to your growing child. If you can find other women who have been through NVP, try drawing on them as another source of strength. While they may admit that they can't do much more for the sufferer than "give her a wet washcloth" (Susan) or "pat her on the back and give her a bag" (Mary), they know what it's like to experience an illness that no sufferer can describe and no nonsufferer seems to believe in. Mary says, "It's not going to be any fun, but you do live through it. . . . Of course, that doesn't help when you're going through it."

Mary offered what is perhaps the best advice overall: to accept rather than continuously combat the apparently unconquerable symptoms of NVP. In my fourth month, my vomiting became predictable enough that I could work out a livable routine. I learned that the first thing to hit my stomach in the morning would immediately come up, but most everything thereafter would stay down. So every morning I began the day with a cup of tea I didn't want—a decoy substance. I would then walk out to the porch (a cool and refreshing change of scene from the bathroom) and throw up over the side. Then I'd go in and eat my breakfast.

Eventually, you too may find ways of working with or around your symptoms so that you can regain some sense of control. Then again, perhaps it's better just to get used to relinquishing control over your life, since your baby will have some ideas about that even after he or she is born. And once the baby comes, remembering your NVP may help you understand what it's like to be helpless, unable to control your body, devastated by hunger, your emotions inextricably bound up with your physical well-being. That's how your baby will feel. Your baby will also throw up a lot. At least you'll be able to sympathize.

2

Headache

MOST WOMEN ENTER PREGNANCY WITH a certain set of expectations, many of which are based on tradition. Despite the shaky foundation of tradition—the vague notion that a thing has always been done in a particular way—it has a surprisingly solid reputation, so solid that violating tradition is something like trying to blast your way through bedrock with a cherry bomb.

If you are having a miserable pregnancy, you are already in violation of the traditional social image of the gestating mother—and not by choice, either, which only increases the difficulty of your role. It is also possible that your pregnancy problems violate a traditional medical view. When that happens, you may have some trouble just convincing your medical practitioner that the problems exist. Once you do, you and your doctor still have to work together to evaluate the problems and agree on how they should be treated, if at all.

According to the traditional view of both neurology and obstetrics, most migraine sufferers experience an improvement of their symptoms in pregnancy. If your experience does not follow this pattern, you may find that tradition has very little to offer, even in the way of recognition of your problem—let alone relief.

Yet the literature is full of cases in which migraine symptoms stayed the same, grew worse, or even appeared for the first time during pregnancy. Doctors even recognize a sudden, unprecedented attack of migraine as a symptom leading to a diagnosis of pregnancy.[1] Clearly, there is room for a lot of variation in how pregnancy influences migraine.

There may not even be so great a difference between the experience of a woman whose pregnancy improves her migraine and a woman whose pregnancy brings migraine on. The migraine–improvement–during–pregnancy contract includes a bit of fine print, which says that the improvement characteristically begins around the end of the first trimester. There seems to be a tendency among medical professionals to discount problems of the first trimester because they last only twelve weeks. However, for the woman suffering these problems, twelve weeks is an excruciating interval, and in no case is relief at the end of that period assured—only traditional.

For Pam, the fact that her migraines improved dramatically in the second trimester did not diminish the painful memories of the first:

> Before I got pregnant I usually had a bad migraine once or twice a month that lasted about two days. It was every month. When I got pregnant, the first three months I had nothing but a headache. It was frustrating because I would not take anything for it for fear of hurting the baby. I must say I took a few Goody's [a headache remedy containing aspirin, acetaminophen, and caffeine] at first because I could not stand it, but I suffered through 99 percent of them. And my headaches were always . . . sick headaches, so there was also nausea with them, but that was common with my headaches previously anyway. I asked the doctor if there was something I could take that would not hurt the baby, and he said no.

Bonnie had experienced migraine only a few times when not pregnant, but had classic migraine with aura in all three of her pregnancies:

> I pretty much dealt with the headaches and didn't discuss them much with the doctor. I just accepted them. I took Tylenol. At first I didn't want to take anything for them, because I didn't like taking medications while pregnant. When the headache became severe I would have to go to bed. There were a few times when I had to leave work [as a physical therapy aide]. I would leave my children at day care and my husband would pick them up.

If you have never experienced a migraine before, the intensity of the symptoms may be alarming. A pounding headache can be accompanied by nausea and vomiting. Light and sound may seem unbearable. Your scalp may feel tender. Other possible symptoms include cold hands and feet, chills, dry mouth, and diarrhea. Prior to the onset of the headache you may experience the "aura" of the classic migraine, which may include visual phenomena such as shimmering points of light, an excited or fearful feeling, tingling or numbness in extremities, or impairment of motor functions or speech.

If you experience an attack of this nature or any significant headache in pregnancy, the first thing to do is visit your doctor. The second thing to do is avoid watching any reruns of "Bewitched," the 1960s television sitcom in which the character of neighbor Gladys Kravytz was apparently drawn from outdated medical writings about the "migraine personality." Gladys was a whiny snoop with one recurring line: "Frank, I'm getting a sick headache." Although fortunately the medical world has abandoned the idea, among the general population there are still those who carry a vague notion that "sick headaches" are some kind of attention-getting mechanism used by hypochondriacs. The fact that migraines tend to be a female complaint only contributes to this myth, at least among those unpleasant types who regard any women's health problem as evidence of mental frailty.

Those types aside, evidence strongly suggests that migraine in women, pregnant or not, is influenced by hormonal factors. While the incidence of migraine in children is divided about equally between boys and girls, it is much greater in adult females (estimates hover at around 19 percent) than in males, with the difference becoming evident at puberty. Further, in women, features of migraine such as frequency and severity tend to vary with fluctuations in hormone levels such as occur with menstruation or the use of oral contraceptives. In fact, more than half of female migraine sufferers note a relationship between migraine attacks and menstruation, with attacks occurring at predictable times in their cycles. Some women experience attacks at no other time.

The timing of menstrual migraine varies from woman to woman but tends to be consistent on an individual basis. One woman may experience attacks during her period; another before; another after; still another in midcycle at ovulation. Since each of these possible peaks is a time of dramatic estrogen fluctuation, the attacks seem to be related in some way to changing estrogen levels. It has been suggested that migraine attacks may be triggered by the withdrawal of estrogens. In keeping with this suggestion, studies show that relief of menstrual migraine most commonly occurs when declining estrogen levels rebound and begin to rise again. This phenomenon could explain why pregnancy more often relieves migraine that is associated with menstruation: Attacks that have been consistently relieved by rising estrogen levels are likely staved off by continued high levels in pregnancy.

Unfashionable though it may be to state that sexual hormones affect behavior, the fact is that steroids such as the estrogens exert a powerful influence throughout body and brain. Brain cells have a strong affinity for estrogens, which bind to them to produce direct effects on the central nervous system. From individual to individual, these neurons vary in their response to produce a symphony of different effects, including modification of the many receptors that allow chemical signaling in the brain. The potential for individual variation is one of the things that makes migraine, even when clearly related to hormone levels, such a complex and unpredictable ailment.

The actual mechanism that produces or relieves migraines has not been established. In fact, there is virtually nothing established in the literature of migraine headache. No pronouncement, no matter how reasonable, appears to have gone unchallenged. Although migraine headaches are described in ancient writings and although doctors have been trying to develop a coherent and incontrovertible migraine model for more than one hundred years, the cause of migraine is still unknown. Even the mechanism that produces the pain remains in dispute, meaning that nobody is completely certain why your head hurts, let alone what sets the headache forces in motion.

However, the majority of authors hold to what is called the *vascular theory of migraine*, which seems to have held up pretty well over the last century. According to this theory, the pain of migraine headache is caused by changes in blood flow to the brain. These changes result first from constriction and then from looseness and expansion of the cerebral arteries. Most doctors believe that excessive dilation of these arteries, with the resulting increased blood flow, produces the throbbing headache of migraine, though exactly why this should be the case is still uncertain. Current theory focuses on connections between the cerebral arteries and the fibers of the trigeminal nerve, which supplies sensation to much of the head and face. Dilation of the blood vessels stimulates these nerve fibers, and the stimulated nerves send signals that the cerebral cortex interprets as pain. It may also be true that the same fibers signal the muscles of the neck, causing tightness and spasm. Some authors have further stated that chemicals released by these nerves provoke even greater dilation and thus painful inflammation around the cerebral arteries.[2]

From this hypothesis regarding mechanism, doctors have attempted to trace backward to the factors stimulating the vascular changes. Believing that they are likely directed by chemical signaling in the brain, researchers have measured levels of the chemical messengers called *neurotransmitters* in migrainous and nonmigrainous subjects. While the evidence suggests that there may be many disturbances of neurotransmission and even that there may be different kinds of migraines produced by different chemical signals, in recent years the weight of research has fallen on the prominent changes in the neurotransmitter *serotonin*.

The serotonergic system has evidently been with us for a long time. Its center lies in the brain stem, the "old" brain that we have in common with the lower orders of animals, and its structure remains remarkably similar as you progress up the evolutionary ladder. It is a system built for powerful influence. Nerve cells in the system are unusually elongated, with the power to carry impulses away from the cell body to distant areas of the brain. What's more, the serotonin released from the cells may not always be restricted to nearby receptors in the usual direction of chemical signaling but may be diffused widely to affect distant tissues.

It is not surprising that such an apparently ancient and influential system should demonstrate effects on some of the body's most basic functions. Among them are sleep, temperature, cardiovascular function, mood, and pain perception. Serotonin works in opposition to *catecholamines*, the neurotransmitters that produce alertness and stress responses. In doing so, serotonin may protect the body from overstimulation or adverse reactions to stress. The result is a dampening of the body's sensitivity to stimuli and a lowering of aggressive responses.

How is this important neurotransmitter related to migraine? No one is sure, but tests seem to demonstrate that there is at least an association between migraine attacks and serotonin. During the course of a migraine attack, levels of serotonin in the blood often fall dramatically. It may be that this lowered level in the blood stimulates a sudden release of serotonin from the brain, because the chemical is self-regulated with a feedback system that signals the brain when blood levels are low. A recent theory of migraine holds that the sudden release of serotonin from the brain activates the "headache pathway" by dilating the blood vessels.[3] It is also possible that low levels of serotonin in the blood render an individual more sensitive to pain by a simultaneous decrease in *B-endorphins*, chemicals involved in decreasing the sensation of pain.

Because of the feedback regulation of serotonin, many migraine therapies are directed at increasing the amount of serotonin available in the blood in order to prevent the sudden release of the chemical from brain cells. As it happens, among the naturally occurring substances associated with higher blood levels of serotonin are the estrogens. Whether estrogens actually stimulate serotonin levels to rise or are associated in some other way is not known, but the parallel increases may be partly responsible for the tendency of migraine, both in the menstrual cycle and in pregnancy, to improve as estrogen levels rise.

However, remember that even if you are lucky enough to experience relief of migraine in pregnancy, it probably won't happen until at least the second trimester. You may also experience a migraine headache for the first time in pregnancy. How might serotonin be associated with migraine in these cases?

There are a number of possibilities. First of all, the serotonergic system seems predisposed to easy disturbance. Persons prone to migraine are often sensitive to certain triggers—foods such as chocolate or cheese, flashing lights, medications, or emotional stress. Somehow, these triggers may stimulate a reaction of the serotonergic system that initiates the attack. Some authors believe that every individual has the potential for a migraine attack, and a sudden, novel combination of triggers could bring on an attack for the first time. In pregnancy, your sensitivity to triggers may be suddenly exaggerated. Just for example, taste and smell can be heightened, especially in the first trimester. (Carol reported that she could barely make it through the produce section of her grocery store without getting woozy from the odors. "I could *smell* the broccoli," she moaned.) Tastes or smells you previously enjoyed suddenly can seem repulsive. It is not a great stretch to imagine that such hypersensitivity to sensory stimulation could translate into increased sensitivity to migraine triggers. The serotonergic system is also sensitive to swings in metabolism and glucose levels, which often occur in pregnancy.

Another possibility involves the relationship of the serotonergic system to the system that produces the catecholamine *norepinephrine*. Levels of the two neurotransmitters seem to rise and fall more or less in concert. Do the apparently low levels of norepinephrine in pregnancy (see Chapter 3) suggest that serotonin levels may sometimes be low as well, stimulating the release of serotonin some authors believe to bring on headache?

Perhaps more provocative than any of these possible connections is the discovery that in rats, human chorionic gonadotropin or HCG—the "pregnancy hormone" whose levels skyrocket from conception throughout the first trimester—stimulates the release of serotonin.[4] If migraine attacks are caused by or in any way related to the sudden release of serotonin, and HCG stimulates that release, it seems logical that women would be intensely vulnerable to migraine attacks in pregnancy, at least in the first trimester.

Further, although headache may be relieved when levels of estrogens are high, apparently those levels must also be stable. The increased incidence of migraine in women using oral contraceptives or estrogen supplements—an effect that has been observed for more than thirty years—may result from unstable estrogen levels.[5] After all, even though the dose may be regular, the body must handle a sudden onslaught of sex steroids each time a pill is taken. Research into the use of oral contraceptives suggests that in some women, the liver (where sex steroids such as the estrogens are broken down) may have difficulty handling the sudden overload of estrogens, which in some women may result in nausea and vomiting. Perhaps in other women, a similar problem with fluctuating estrogen levels produces migraine. In the first trimester of pregnancy, the liver is bombarded with sex steroids far above the usual amounts. Perhaps this explains the utter chaos that some women perceive in their bodies in these early months, a chaos that tends to resolve at least partially sometime in the second trimester, as the liver adjusts to the new hormone load. Given the condition of the internal environment, it seems likely that a woman in early pregnancy qualifies for the instability of hormone levels believed to be associated with increased incidence of migraine. Notably, too, the disturbance of liver function in early pregnancy may result in a decreased ability to metabolize tryptophan–which just happens to be the substance from which serotonin is manufactured.

In another interesting possible connection between serotonin and first-trimester pregnancy symptoms, it has been suggested that because the body stores serotonin in cells within the intestine, vomiting may be a defense mechanism the body uses to raise serotonin levels in the blood.[6] Perhaps this defense might be employed in pregnancy.

The estrogens influence other substances that have shown an association with migraine attacks. Among them are *prostaglandins*, fatty acids whose production by the uterine lining is triggered by the release of the neurotransmitter norepinephrine and influenced by the estrogens and progesterone. Rising levels of prostaglandins inhibit the further release of norepinephrine so that transmission slows along certain pathways. This slowed transmission has a significant effect on the perception of pain, because the body's natural pain control mechanisms depend on these pathways and the presence of norepinephrine. So powerful is the influence of prostaglandins over normal pain control that even morphine becomes less effective in their presence.

Even as they decrease the body's natural ability to cope with pain, the prostaglandins promote inflammation of nerves and sensitize pain receptors. Studies have demonstrated that prostaglandins can also stimulate two of the most painful symptoms associated with the menstrual cycle: uterine contractions and headache. Subjects in one study received certain prostaglandins through IVs and came down with whopping headaches and abdominal cramps. In another study–the sort for which you hope the subjects were handsomely compensated–women with painful periods and menstrual migraine were tapped for blood samples during their periods, then later reinfused with that blood. The reinfusion stimulated the same symptoms experienced in menstruation, headache among them.[7]

In a number of animal species, prostaglandins apparently prepare the uterus for implantation, and pregnancy cannot be achieved if synthesis of prostaglandins is blocked. This does not appear to be the case for humans–in fact, prostaglandins administered in early pregnancy induce abortion–but there may be an important role, as yet undiscovered, for prostaglandins in the establishment of a human pregnancy. It has been demonstrated that before implantation embryos can produce prostaglandins, which may be involved in the beginning steps of the development of the embryo. Thus prostaglandins may be in the maternal circulation but perhaps directed away from the uterine lining. (In some nonprimate species, the embryo appears actually to have this ability of redirection.)[8] It does not seem entirely farfetched to suggest that prostaglandins may play a role in the headache of early pregnancy, as they do in menstrual migraine.

While migraine appearing for the first time in pregnancy most often occurs in the first trimester, dramatic presentations of first-time migraine have also been recorded in the last few months, when hormone levels presumably have stabilized. In such cases, it is worth considering that not all doctors attribute migraine pain solely to vascular dilation in the brain. Mechanical irritation of nerves is another possibility cited in some papers. An example of how this may occur might explain the connection sometimes observed between migraine and sleep. Neck movements in sleep can irritate nerves, causing muscle spasms that draw the vertebrae of the neck closer together, which both pinches the nerves passing through the vertebrae and forces the discs between vertebrae to bulge outward. The resulting pain may cause further neck movement, causing further pain, and so on until the input from the inflamed nerves triggers the headache pathway. The patient awakens with a whopping migraine.[9]

In late pregnancy, posture changes can cause extreme irritation of the nerves around the cervical (neck) vertebrae. Many doctors believe that cervical disc problems are often responsible for the symptoms of carpal tunnel syndrome many women experience in pregnancy. It certainly seems possible that irritation of other nerves by misaligned cervical discs could be at least partially responsible for unprecedented headache pain.

Reports of late-pregnancy, first-time migraines often feature dramatic symptoms such as difficult speech, blurred vision, and even weakness or numbness in one side of the body. Doctors stress that pounding headache with any of these symptoms can be a sign of a serious problem apart from migraine and should be thoroughly evaluated. On the other hand, many of the reported cases have turned up no abnormalities in any neurological testing, providing no answers whatsoever to the mystery of sudden-onset classic migraine in late pregnancy.

The fact is that during pregnancy, the body's internal environment is altered in so many ways that researchers may never be able to pinpoint one precipitating factor in the onset or worsening of migraine. Apart from any hormonal disturbances, there are dramatic changes in nutritional needs, metabolism, fluid exchange, the immune system, and the cardiovascular system. When you consider that the root cause of migraine has yet to be established, it seems almost impossible that a complete understanding of pregnancy-related migraine lies anywhere on the road ahead.

Feeling Better

Fortunately, there are some treatments available that are safe in pregnancy and may prove effective for you. For the most part, these treatments are not pharmacological. In pregnancy, treating migraine with medication is a difficult business. The most common prescription for relief of migraine, ergotamine tartrate, is one of a class of drugs (ergot alkaloids) not recommended in pregnancy because they may promote abortion by increasing uterine motor activity. In fact, if you are a migraine sufferer taking regular doses of this or any drug to prevent attacks, you should discuss with your doctor the possibility of discontinuing the medication. Even aspirin is to be avoided. Doctors suggest limiting headache medications to acetaminophen (for example Tylenol), which unfortunately may provide little relief in severe migraine attacks. If you do take acetaminophen, one doctor suggests taking it dissolved in a warm, sweetened beverage to increase its absorption and effectiveness.[10] Be aware, however, that overuse of any pain medication may result in a rebound effect that can increase the frequency of headache. The medical literature notes that pain medication taken more than two or three days a week for six to eight weeks puts the user at risk for rebound headaches.[11]

Some "extra-strength" headache remedies combine aspirin or acetaminophen with caffeine, which relieves some headaches by constricting blood vessels in the brain. Many women ingest caffeine in small amounts during their pregnancies with a daily cup of coffee (80 to 100 milligrams) or tea (50 to 80 milligrams); the amount contained in one dose of pain reliever ranges from 16.25 milligrams (one Goody's tablet) to 65 milligrams (one Bayer Select caplet).

Outside of pharmacology, the array of possible treatments for headache is rather large. Some may be effective both in reducing frequency of headaches and in stopping them when they do begin. Anything that promotes good physical health and reduces stress may prove effective in both regards. For this reason, physical medicine (chiropractic, physical therapy), exercise, diet modifications, herbal medicine, and techniques for promoting relaxation (biofeedback, hypnosis) are worth considering as part of your anti-headache regimen.

Physical medicine. Both the mainstream (physical therapy) and alternative (chiropractic, acupressure, acupuncture) varieties of physical or manipulative medicine may be one of the great untapped resources in headache management. Dr. Charles Theisler strongly recommends chiropractic manipulation, citing success rates of 72 to 90 percent in various studies. Interestingly, while the cervical vertebrae are often the primary focus of such treatment, Theisler further notes that a small percentage of migraine patients apparently require manipulation of the sacroiliac joints for sustained headache relief.[12] A number of recent studies on backache in pregnancy have found problems with the sacroiliac joints in pregnant subjects (see Chapter 11).

If you are hesitant about chiropractic treatments, at least consider the possible benefits of massage. Though probably of little benefit as a long-term treatment, massage may be very comforting and helpful during a headache. Warm your neck and shoulder area first with hot packs, as it may increase the benefits of the massage.

Pam consulted a physical therapist for exercises to help control her migraine pain in pregnancy. A typesetter for a book publisher, Pam found the exercises not only helpful for headaches but generally refreshing to perform at intervals during a day of typing at the video terminal, since the exercises focused on relieving neck and shoulder strain. One exercise was to grasp her chair with one hand and lean her head slowly to the opposite side, hold for a few seconds to stretch the neck muscles, then repeat with the opposite hand. The therapist also helped Pam adjust her chair and desk for prevention of strain. If you spend a lot of time in front of a computer, this kind of service from a physical therapist might prove especially helpful for you. If your OB or another medical doctor refers you to the therapist, insurance will usually cover the therapist's services. (A doctor's referral is not necessarily required as insurance company practices vary.)

Posture-related devices. A cervical collar at night may help by preventing excessive neck movement.[13] Given the problems pregnant women tend to have with night backache (see Chapter 11) and nighttime exaggeration of carpal tunnel syndrome (Chapter 12), such a device seems well worth trying, as it may help prevent these other nerve problems apparently related to lying down.

Moving from top to bottom, you should also give some thought to your footwear. If you have not already abandoned your high-heeled shoes, do so now. The posture problems related to high heels are certainly capable of irritating cervical nerves. In addition, assuming you cannot wear your running shoes 100 percent of the time, inside your sensible office flats you might consider using shoe inserts to reduce shock to the spine. Inserts of Sorbothane and other shock-absorbing materials are available over-the-counter at drugstores and sporting goods stores. You may have to experiment with different brands to find a fit that feels right. Podiatrists and some physical therapists can also measure you for custom shoe inserts to correct different leg length or mechanical problems of the hip or spine.

Exercise. Exercise has sometimes been reported effective in migraine therapy, both in preventing attacks and in cutting them short when they occur. The exact beneficial action is not known, but among the possibilities are

- *that because exercise causes painless dilation of the scalp blood vessels, regular exercise might somehow accustom these vessels to dilation so that dilation is no longer painful;*

- *that exercise, which has been demonstrated to increase the body's pain threshold, might increase a migraine sufferer's levels of endorphins, counteracting the deficiency seen in many migraine patients;*

- *that regular exercise may provoke sustained increases in serotonin levels; and*

- *that exercise might promote more moderate release or effective use of catecholamines, the neurotransmitters whose release inspires a counteractive release of serotonin.*[14]

In any case, moderate, regular exercise (see Appendix for guidelines) may help reduce the frequency or intensity of headaches and may even help stop an attack if you can get out and walk when you feel a headache coming on. One benefit of exercise at the beginning of an attack may be to redistribute blood flow from your head to your limbs. However, some people report that exercise actually seems to bring on headaches. If you are exercising and feel a headache coming on, you may be reacting to an overload of oxygen. Slow down–try not to stop entirely, since cooling down is important in keeping the headache away–and hold a paper bag over your nose and mouth for a moment, breathing in and out of the bag. You will be breathing the carbon dioxide you exhale, which will counteract the extra oxygen.[15] Do this only briefly; you should feel the changes quickly, especially if you were feeling dizzy or lightheaded.

Relaxation. Various relaxation techniques are used in the treatment of migraine. One popular therapy is biofeedback training, a stress management technique that helps the body to "unlearn" harmful stress responses. Biofeedback training includes the use of instruments that measure impulses generated within the body as reactions to stress. The instruments translate these impulses into auditory or visual signals that provide the patient with a clear picture of how her body reacts to certain stimuli. With this picture in mind, the patient is trained to prevent these reactions with relaxation techniques.

Hypnotherapy, which also involves relaxation, is well established as an effective treatment for chronic pain, including the pain of migraine attacks. A visit to a hypnotherapist might involve a discussion of your pain, agreement on an appropriate suggestion that your therapist will offer when you are in the trance state, and the induction itself. The induction is a process of focusing and relaxation. (To ascertain that you have reached the desired level of relaxation, your therapist may offer a suggestion, such as that one of your arms is growing so light that it will float up toward the ceiling. You will be perfectly aware during this time and will likely get a good giggle at yourself as your arm responds.) Once you are in the trance state, your therapist will use the agreed-upon suggestion regarding relief of your pain, then bring you out of the trance. The more often you do this, the better it is likely to work, so your therapist may also teach you some self-hypnosis skills for strengthening the suggestion through repetition. Some therapists may help you by recording your sessions on audio cassettes.

Dietary changes. Because certain foods are demonstrated triggers of migraine in sensitive persons, dietary modifications may be an important step toward preventing headaches. Among the most common sensitivities are cheese, chocolate, and foods containing monosodium glutamate, such as Chinese food. Beyond those, individual sensitivities might encompass everything from wheat or corn to avocados. If you can connect your headaches to any food or group of foods, by all means find a way to eliminate those foods from your diet. A book on food allergies might be useful in helping you determine sensitivities and make substitutions.

Whatever you can eat, eat it immediately. Hunger can produce headaches in the stablest of bodies, and you, being pregnant, do not have the stablest of bodies. It is best not to allow yourself even to get hungry, but if you do, find food as quickly as possible. Nonsweet, stabilizing fare will protect you longer from blood sugar swings, but ending with a bite or two of something very sweet might enhance protection against headache.

Herbs. Certain herbs have proved effective for many people in relieving migraine, but not all of them are safe in pregnancy. For example, feverfew, whose effectiveness as a headache treatment has won it notice in the medical journals, is also used to promote menstrual flow and should not be taken by pregnant women. Mint teas are apparently safe and very pleasant. On the whole, make use of herbs, but regard their actions seriously; there is often more than folklore behind them. Research herbs, even those in charmingly packaged teas from the grocery store, as much as you can before using them.

Incidentally, you don't have to ingest herbs to enjoy their beneficial effects. Application of herbal compresses or inhalation of steam from various herbal brews may help relax you or clear away unpleasant odors that can trigger migraines. Again, look in herbal manuals for suggestions.

Pressure devices. Putting pressure on the scalp, with the fingers or with something wound tightly around the head, is a remedy most migraine sufferers discover on their own. A physician in Sacramento[16] has developed and patented a device that works on this principle: an elastic band whose tightness is adjusted with Velcro closures. The device includes flat rubber discs that slip under the band to increase pressure on specific areas without tightening the band too much elsewhere. Although some patients in this doctor's care could not use the band because of scalp tenderness (not an uncommon phenomenon with migraine), many others found that the device significantly alleviated their pain. This device is available through Self-Care at 1-800-345-3371.

Cold therapy. Ice packs are also a common treatment, and there are now devices available that provide this cold therapy without the bother of drippy ice bags sliding off your head. A medical journal recently carried an ad for Cold Hats, which look something like the bonnet attachments of old-fashioned hairdryers but could make up in relief for what they lack in sex appeal. These are available through Mason and Mason Engineering, 3915 Rosewood, Longview CA 98632, 1-800-594-7122. You could also check your local drugstore for cold-wrap devices.

Sleep rationing. The relationship between sleep and migraine varies from person to person. Some migraine sufferers find that brief naps help to ward off oncoming headaches, and many others find that sleep is inevitably the final stage of an attack. However, some migraine patients have found that oversleeping seems to trigger attacks. Recently, a physician described in the journal *Headache* how he controlled his own nocturnal migraines by restricting himself to four hours of sleep a night supplemented with an afternoon nap of up to an hour.[17] He based his system on the findings of a physician named M. Gans, whose system of "sleep-rationing" reduced the frequency of migraine attacks in his patients. This system involved not only reduction of sleep hours but the lightening of sleep stages by having the patients touched frequently throughout the night. Thus the patients were less likely to sink into the deep sleep stages that have been associated with migraine in some persons.[18]

Interestingly, women in late stages of pregnancy tend to become unwilling participants in a sleep reduction regimen. Studies suggest that the deepest stages of sleep become decreased or disappear altogether in the third trimester (see Chapter 5). As for overall sleep time, it doesn't take a body of medical research (though the research has been done all the same) to tell us that women in the last months of pregnancy lose a lot more sleep than their nonpregnant acquaintances thanks to backache, leg cramps, heartburn, and bathroom trips as well as to undetermined but apparently hormonally regulated mechanisms. Conversely, the first trimester often brings great fatigue, which the more fortunate may combat with long naps—which are associated with migraine in some people—or longer hours in bed at night. It is at least worth wondering whether these common effects of pregnancy may in some way relate to the relief or occurrence of migraine. It may even be worth experimenting with your sleep time, though it is hard to imagine a pregnant woman willingly rationing those precious hours.

Even if the headaches you experience in pregnancy are not associated with migraine symptoms, any of the therapies suggested in this chapter is well worth trying. Even ordinary tension headaches may be produced by mechanisms similar to those of migraine attacks, perhaps at a lesser point on a continuum of response and pain.

The acclaimed neurologist and author Oliver Sacks, in his book *Migraine: Understanding a Common Disorder,*[19] offers additional insight into migraine by considering it from the perspective of evolutionary biology. How might the migraine headache have developed in the human species? Where does such a monstrous affliction fit in a picture of evolution as a process of positive adaptations–that is, a process in which the individuals bearing a certain trait tend to prosper and reproduce because that trait conveys an advantage? In considering this question, Sacks proposes a concept of migraine that casts a new light on many of the strange symptoms of pregnancy.

First of all, Sacks builds his argument on the relationship, amply demonstrated over decades of research, between migraine attacks and stress. Some researchers have postulated that persons prone to migraine are hypersensitive to changes in levels of neurotransmitters and that the resulting instability of neurotransmission impairs their ability to adapt to change, whether within their bodies or their environment.[20] But Sacks disputes the assumption that migraine attacks represent an impaired stress response. Instead, he explores the possibility that a migraine attack is itself a form of response–not the adrenaline-rush, "fight or flight" reaction most of us imagine as a response to threat, but another kind of response equally common in nature, the *passive protective reaction.*

As Sacks points out, examples of the passive protective reaction are present in many species. Each involves some kind of immobility, and often an accompanying secretory response. A rabbit freezes at the sight of an approaching dog; a frightened dog may vomit in the presence of threat; a possum plays dead; a chameleon frantically changes color (an internal secretory response) to convince the potential attacker that he's simply not there. These reactions are the animal's attempt to somehow take itself, if not out of harm's way, at least out of its notice.

Sacks notes that human beings are entirely capable of dramatic passive protective responses, including fainting and narcolepsy. Within this repertoire of reponse he lists the migraine attack, which is characterized by "passivity, stillness, and immobilization."[21] A person suffering a migraine is forced by pain, lethargy, and perhaps intolerance of light and sound to withdraw from his or her environment and often falls asleep before the migraine is relieved. Sacks maintains that the triggering of migraine by stress may represent a passive protective reaction developed over our evolutionary course. Contributing to that development, as humans became more social–and so perhaps required new withdrawal reactions–they also became more complex in neurological development, allowing new responses, such (perhaps) as migraine, to become elaborated in the cerebral cortex.

Within this concept, other pregnancy complaints seem to take on new meaning. Depression, nausea, and vomiting all fit Sacks's description of passive protective responses. At a time when society expects excitement and vigor and presses in on you with its desire to share the happy event, your body may be crying, "Threat! Threat!" and collapsing like a possum in the shadow of a predator. In fact, society's enthusiasm for pregnancy seems to allow no room for what your body instinctively understands: The sudden derangement of your internal environment represents a state of high stress demanding protective, adaptive responses for the sake of survival. In this light, it is interesting to reconsider the hoary theory that a pregnancy symptom like vomiting represents the mother's unconscious rejection of the baby. This theory makes sense if you can think of an unconscious act as something the body does to maintain itself, independent of any effort of intellect–breathing, for example. Your body may, with perfect justification, perceive pregnancy as a threat to its accustomed state, quite apart from however you may feel about it. As evidence, consider the fact that pregnancy symptoms exactly of this passive protective nature often occur before the mother is aware of the pregnancy. Once pregnancy is confirmed, powerful psychosocial factors may also contribute to the stress, increasing the strength of the response.

Perhaps the single most difficult thing about miserable pregnancy symptoms is how they separate, sometimes with ruthless force, the thinking, feeling you from your physical self. For nine months you may have to live in a body that is out of sync with your intellectual and emotional responses to pregnancy. If evolution is responsible, then survival of the fittest just isn't all it's cracked up to be. Nevertheless, survival is your goal. Talk as much as you can to other women who have really been there. They have lived to walk among the fittest again. So will you.

3

Mood Disorders

"I STAYED DEPRESSED DURING MY WHOLE second pregnancy," said Barbara. "I did." She went on:

> Of course I felt better during my second trimester, physically. But I was so uncomfortable my third trimester. I was just not a happy pregnant woman. And I remember standing in the kitchen sometimes and crying, and telling my husband, "I just want you to understand how I feel. . . ."
>
> I knew when I had the child I would feel differently about it, but I was in the *now*—stuck in that big, uncomfortable body. And a sad heart.

Women are brave. There is simply no other way to explain our willingness, generation after generation, to create pregnancies and carry them to their logical conclusions. Deciding to bear a child means opening oneself completely to physical and emotional experiences that are unpredictable and often uncontrollable. It also means a lifetime commitment to an experience about which one has only the faintest of clues.

To face these challenges, pregnancy demands a complete rearrangement of a woman's psychological landscape. At the same time, the biochemical environment of her body is thrown into chaos. Small wonder that among the most common complaints of pregnancy are emotional disruptions ranging from mood swings to full-blown depression.

Preexisting Depression

Among the bravest women, then, are those who enter pregnancy with a preexisting tendency toward depression. These women have known what it is to live with feelings of worthlessness, guilt, and helplessness that seem to come out of nowhere and take up permanent residence, feeding bizarrely on themselves until their magnitude threatens to choke off the life of their victim. Almost without exception, women who have suffered bouts of this kind of depression describe the possibility of repeat performances as frightening, even terrifying. Many make use of medication to forestall this possibility—medication that, for ethical reasons, cannot be scientifically studied for safety in human pregnancy. Yet these women, too, make the choice to enter a state of biological upheaval widely known to produce or exacerbate depressive symptoms. It is an act of phenomenal courage.

How does a woman face it? Sometimes she researches medication, as Barbara describes:

> We asked around before we even got pregnant for the first time, because my husband had been working with some prenatal people. And we talked to the OB-GYN in my first pregnancy about whether or not I should be on the Prozac. And he said, because there had been really few studies, he didn't have enough evidence to say I should get off it . . . but I guess he'd seen enough women on it that he felt the risk was pretty slim. The question was important because prior to my getting pregnant the depression had been severe. I was pretty scared of the depression. And I didn't really have any idea, of course, what the pregnancy would be like. I was a little apprehensive about taking Prozac . . . but both the doctor and I felt that the alternative of severe depression would benefit neither me nor the baby.

Sometimes she reaches for hope where she can find it, in a word, a tone of voice—even, says Barbara, in a rationalization:

> My OB was reassuring enough—I mean, he dealt with complicated pregnancies all the time, and he saw people on all kinds of drugs. And I guess I did some rationalization too, thinking, "He's seen people on everything, because he's a prenatal specialist, and so if this seems minor to him, and I don't detect any concern in his voice, then I'm gonna take his permission and run with it."

Sometimes, like Barbara, she cries:

> I think the fact that my second child was unexpected was a big factor in my depression at that time. Theoretically we had been thinking about another child, but we certainly weren't down to the planning stages. And the weekend that I found out I was pregnant again was the weekend of a big blizzard. And talk about feeling

> trapped. I sat on this couch and cried, and cried, and cried. . . . I felt so trapped. Trapped with a not quite two-and-a-half-year-old. I can't even remember all the feelings I had. I felt angry. That was the predominant feeling, being trapped and angry and depressed, and I sat on that couch—I can remember it so vividly—that whole weekend. Just crying, and crying, and crying.

In the face of this kind of bravery and this depth of suffering, it is appalling to think that most pregnant women with emotional disorders receive little more than a pat on the hand and a patronizing reminder like, "Pregnancy is an emotional time for everyone." Most people would readily agree that pregnancy is a stressful experience, but few understand the physical stresses involved and how they can affect the emotions, even if you have no prior history of emotional disorder. In turn, emotions can have a pronounced effect on a woman's ability to function in everyday life.

Depression is the most common mood disorder in both pregnant and nonpregnant people, and the symptoms of depression strike at the very heart of the sufferer's ability to carry out the tasks of work and family living: inability to concentrate and make decisions, withdrawal, lack of initiative, inactivity, disturbances in sleep and eating. On top of all this, the pregnant woman may suffer physical symptoms such as intense nausea and vomiting, backache, migraine, fatigue, and other complaints. It is impossible that her daily life should go unaffected.

"My performance at work became riddled with anxiety," wrote Louise, a lifelong sufferer of depression whose pregnancies were also complicated with nausea, vomiting, and other illness. "I coped by being sick and eventually quitting."

Dawn M. suffered similar disruptions without even understanding their cause—with the same result:

> Not knowing I was pregnant, my job seemed to be becoming more demanding and stressful. With all of the changes I was going through (sleeplessness, indigestion, nausea, headaches off and on) I chalked it up to stress. My job became too much for me to cope with, so I quit.

Colleen described how pregnancy-related depression affected her family relationships:

> The way I was feeling, I can't even describe it, except that I didn't want any man around me. "I don't need you, you got me pregnant," you know. It's almost anger, too, I think: "Look what I'm going through." My first trimester was really hard on everyone. Not only my husband, but my family. I mean, I was very irritating to be around. I talked to the women that really know me. I told

them how I was feeling, and they kept reassuring me that it was just a temporary thing, and I was like, "No, no. You don't understand." So I did reach out for help, and people were telling me stuff, but I wasn't believing them.

Like Colleen–indeed, like nearly every woman interviewed for this book who described her emotional state in pregnancy–Linda M. noted the difficulty of distinguishing between reactions to hormones and reactions to the circumstances of her life.

In the middle trimester I was quite emotional. I am not normally a big crier, but I cried a lot. It was hard for me to judge whether my reactions were due to hormones or to some other very real things going on in my life.

The fact is that it is not always possible to separate the two. The psychiatric profession now recognizes a biological basis for many emotional disorders. A disturbance in the biochemical environment of the brain can affect psychological functioning in ways that are well beyond the control of the individual. At the same time, confusing the picture even further, it has been suggested that psychological functioning shapes brain biochemistry. To understand how interior and exterior circumstances work together to produce the emotional experience of pregnancy, one must consider, first, the biochemical processes that influence personality and emotion, and second, the real stressors of pregnancy and how they might affect those processes.

The Biology of Personality

Women just now entering their childbearing years may not recall the days when high school home ec classes included lectures on improving one's personality, but those of us who fared badly in the subject should take heart. Our low scores did not necessarily reflect a lack of attention in class. Within the last twenty-five years, researchers have focused on personality as the product of brain functions that are far beyond the purview of even the most dedicated home ec teacher. In particular, recent research has turned away from a concentration of electrical signaling to focus instead on brain activity as a chemical process. As seems to be the case with most brain research, each discovery in this field has led only to more complex questions. Once it was determined that most of the communication in the central nervous system (CNS) takes place through chemical actions, researchers concentrated on identifying the chemicals called neurotransmitters and tracing their pathways of message transfer across the surface of the brain and throughout the CNS.

Just as this research was falling into place, evidence began to suggest that other substances were also capable of affecting communication between neurons. Perhaps most interesting where pregnant women are concerned is that hormones appear to be among those substances. In many recent studies, patients suffering mood disturbances such as depression have demonstrated abnormal levels of or abnormal response to certain hormones. Significantly, similar alterations of neuroendocrine function are associated with pregnancy.

Today, it is evident that chemical signaling in the CNS involves legions of messengers, chemicals of all sorts whose interactions are, to put it mildly, imperfectly understood. Further, those interactions are likely influenced by genetic and environmental factors, both of which may actually affect the formation of the pathways along which neurotransmitters travel.

How does disturbed function of neurotransmitters lead to emotional disorders? While researchers have a long way to go toward answering that question, one possibility is that abnormalities of neurotransmission produce changes in the brain's use of glucose, its primary fuel. With sophisticated imaging technology, researchers are able to trace the metabolism of glucose throughout the brain. They have also found that changes in that metabolism are closely associated with changes in cerebral circulation. Studies of both depressed and manic patients have found abnormalities in both metabolism and circulation in the brain. Perhaps these are among the responses to neurotransmitter disturbance that are manifested in the symptoms of emotional disorder.

It is evident, then, that a person with a mood disorder may be suffering the influence of many stressors, among them hormonal, metabolic, environmental, and social. As many of these stressors are also characteristic of pregnancy, it is hardly surprising that emotional disturbance is common among pregnant women.

What is uncommon, apparently, is the inclination of health professionals to take this disturbance seriously or to invest many research dollars in understanding the causes. The available literature on emotional disorders in pregnancy is rather scanty, and much of what does exist is thirty or forty years old. This may be another place where the women's movement backfired for its pregnant members. Thirty or forty years ago, it seems, people more readily assumed that pregnancy predisposed women to psychological disorders. A 1959 mental health publication of the U.S. government contained the following observation:

> If a psychologist takes a Rorschach on a pregnant woman, he may come to you and say, "This woman is very ill." And if you give him ten pregnant women to test, he would probably say, "They are all very ill." If you say, "No, they're just pregnant," he will answer, "But

look at this picture; there are very strong suggestions of schizophrenic process here. The defenses have crumpled."[1]

Regrettably, in the popular culture, such observations degenerated into demeaning stereotypes of hysterical women suffering "female troubles"—exactly the sort of stereotype that women have spent the last few decades fighting to eliminate. The unfortunate consequence is a backlash assumption that pregnant women who do suffer emotional disturbance are falling victim to stereotypical roles from which they could release themselves with the proper attitude and education.

The first step to correcting this assumption is careful consideration of the research that has been performed on disordered mood—especially depression, the most common manifestation—in pregnancy.

It is well established that over a lifetime, a woman is more likely than a man to suffer depression. In childhood, boys and girls suffer depression about equally, but beginning at adolescence, the higher prevalence is among females, which suggests an association with the reproductive hormones. Those hormones have been found to exert a significant influence on brain function, affecting the biochemical environment of the nerve cells and thus influencing how signals are transmitted through the brain and body. They also influence circadian rhythms, the "clock cycles" of the body, which are likewise associated with mood disturbances.

Any time hormones are present in unusual concentrations, an individual is at risk for emotional changes. This effect has been observed in conditions such as Cushing's syndrome, in which excessive steroid levels result in initial euphoria that eventually turns to mood swings and depression. It is also, of course, widely observed in healthy, normal women going through just about all significant stages of reproductive life. Among these stages, a psychiatry text lists puberty, postpartum depression, and menopause—but, inexplicably, omits pregnancy.[2] Nevertheless, in view of the demonstrated emotional effects of sex steroids, it seems impossible that they should not have a major influence on the mood and behavior of the pregnant woman.

The few bold souls who have ventured to discuss mental states in pregnancy seem to agree on one thing: The subject is poorly studied. Estimating the incidence of pregnancy-related depression is difficult, partly because of the lack of studies and partly because existing research is not consistent in its measurement of psychological disturbance. Estimates on the prevalence of clinical depression in pregnancy range up to about 50 percent, with some depressive symptoms showing up even more frequently, especially when reported by the woman herself rather than evaluated by the researcher. Up to 68 percent of pregnant women have reported inexplicable crying spells, and cases of the blues have been reported by as many as 84 percent.

The most consistent numbers for the occurrence of clinical depression in pregnancy fall between 16 and 18 percent. Many of these figures have been drawn from studies in the United States and several European countries; however, similar figures have been reported from tribal societies in Africa, despite the Western fancy that tribal women enjoy carefree, "natural" pregnancies unencumbered by the psychosomatic difficulties engendered by our society.

Further problems stem from the fact that these estimates encompass only *clinical* depression—that is, depression severe enough to require treatment. A recent study from California points out that no studies have focused on the occurrence of depressive *symptoms* in pregnancy. The psychiatric profession uses a set of guidelines, involving a checklist of eight symptoms that must be experienced under specific conditions, to diagnose clinical depression. The California study notes that while only 5 percent of their subjects met these criteria, 50 percent of all subjects reported high levels of at least three of the symptoms on the checklist, especially anger, fatigue, anxiety, and worry. The California researchers speculate that large numbers of women may experience a pattern of depressive symptoms unique to childbearing yet not falling within the guidelines for clinical depression. The researchers use the term *dysphoria*, a sense of ill-being, to draw a distinction between this pattern and clinical depression.[3]

Except where pregnancy is concerned, the connection between hormones and behavioral changes has received a great deal of study. Of course the female body lends itself to this kind of research, with its pronounced and predictable fluctuations in hormone levels. It is a fairly simple matter to compare these levels with the results of psychological tests or interviews gathered at appropriate times in the menstrual cycle and use these comparisons to make educated guesses relating mood and behavior to hormone levels.

Sufferers of premenstrual syndrome would laugh at the idea that anyone needs test tubes and inkblots to prove a connection between the menstrual cycle and mood. However, some studies suggest that even in women reporting none of the marked emotional changes that characterize PMS—such as sudden mood changes, anger or irritability, depression, or lack of interest in normal activities—the brain behaves differently at different points in the menstrual cycle. In a pair of studies[4] a group of sixteen spontaneously cycling women and sixteen women on oral contraceptives underwent regular hormone measurements, EEGs (readings of brain electrical activity), and psychological performance tests throughout their cycles. The women with spontaneous cycles displayed brain wave patterns different from those of women on oral contraceptives. In the OC nonusers, there were greater differences between certain frequencies and significant accelerations in some patterns during the luteal (postovulation) phase of the cycle. The accelerations dropped off suddenly one to two days before the menstrual period. The women on oral contraceptives did not display any such accelerations, except for a slight acceleration right before their periods when they discontinued the contraceptives in order to bring on menstruation. Overall, the highs and lows of brain waves seen in the OC nonusers seem to have been smoothed out in those using oral contraceptives.

On all performance tests, the women with spontaneous cycles significantly outperformed the contraceptive users in both speed and accuracy. The difference in performance widened as the OC nonusers neared their menstrual periods. The authors of the study noted that progesterone peaks seemed to correlate with high levels of speed and accuracy. However, the best performances of all were recorded one to two days before menstruation, when progesterone would have declined sharply. Thus it is difficult to say exactly how progesterone relates to brain activity in women with spontaneous cycles. Perhaps it is more significant to focus on the users of oral contraceptives, who not only were outperformed but failed to show any of the improvements in performance that were so pronounced in OC nonusers over the course of their cycles. Perhaps continually elevated levels of sex steroids tend to smooth out certain peaks and accelerations of brain waves that are necessary for full alertness and reactivity. If this is true in the use of oral contraceptives, what are the implications for pregnant women?

Arguing further for a connection between reproductive hormones and brain function are the widespread reports of depression associated with oral contraceptive use. Within a few years of the birth control pill's commercial introduction in the early 1960s, medical journals were publishing studies on mood changes in its users. The high doses of estrogens and progesterone in the first contraceptive pills produced some alarming effects. One woman suffered an acute schizophrenic episode when she discontinued use of the oral contraceptive she had been taking. Her symptoms disappeared when she went back on the pill but returned when her doctor substituted a placebo. Many other women reported moderate to severe depression. Some sought psychoanalysis and were found to have no other factor beyond the use of the pill that seemed related to their depressive symptoms, which included lethargy, disinterest in their usual pursuits, and a significant decrease in sex drive.[5] Many women discontinued their use of the pill to relieve these symptoms.

Naturally, the pharmaceutical companies quickly went to work on new formulas for their offerings. By lowering the doses of hormones, they succeeded in reducing (but not eliminating) mood changes. The oral contraceptives in use today contain the lowest possible doses for effective contraception. Still, depressive symptoms are a common side effect.

Researchers have pursued several explanations for this effect, including the predictable female hysteria line (which in this case holds that depression is caused by such factors as confusion about the maternal role and guilt over using contraceptives). In 1988, a study of 1,131 pairs of twins blasted through this line by demonstrating a clear genetic influence in the incidence of psychiatric reactions to oral contraceptives.[6] This finding is consistent with the well-established understanding that genetics help to determine which individuals are most susceptible to psychiatric disorders. Similarly, genes play a role in individual reactions to drugs, whose metabolism and excretion (and thus effect on the body) can vary widely from person to person.

The researchers in this study found that genetic susceptibility to depression from OC use is apparently independent of a predisposition to non-drug-induced depression. (It is also independent of factors predisposing women to weight gain or swelling from OCs, a finding that neatly disposes of the idea that women with OC-related depression are really just feeling gloomy about putting on weight.)

It may be that OCs produce depression at least partly by depleting the vitamin B_6 in the liver. B_6 is an important component in the metabolism of the amino acid *tryptophan* into the mood-influencing neurotransmitter serotonin. Thus oral contraceptives may create a serotonin deficiency, a circumstance long associated with depressive symptoms.

This is not the only time the liver has been implicated in problems related to oral contraceptives. Some researchers believe that nausea and vomiting, other side effects some women suffer, are the result of the liver's inability to metabolize a sudden onslaught of sex steroids. Interestingly, women suffering nausea and vomiting with contraceptive use are highly likely to experience the same symptoms in pregnancy, perhaps because of the same problem with metabolism in the liver. (See Chapter 1.) Perhaps OC-related depression might show a similar association with depression in pregnancy.

Other neurotransmitters besides serotonin have been linked to mood maintenance and disruption. One hypothesis relates mood to the body's use and supply of catecholamines, the neurotransmitters epinephrine and norepinephrine. These exist in fibers in the central nervous system, are produced by the adrenal glands, and are concentrated at sites in the brain. Catecholamines are produced in response to stress—any activity or influence that requires extra attentiveness or energy. A stressor might be a physical activity such as exercise, a mental task, or an instance in which the body's normally balanced interior environment is suddenly out of kilter, as when blood sugar levels become too low (hypoglycemia). Producing a certain level of alertness in the body and brain, catecholamines stimulate the heart, increase oxygen consumption and heat production, and can cause contractions of smooth muscle tissue including the uterine wall.

Excess production of catecholamines may represent a threat to pregnancy. Some animal studies have linked increased catecholamine levels to premature uterine contractions and decreased uterine blood flow. Rodent studies suggest that catecholamines and their metabolism are intricately (though as yet indecipherably) linked with reproductive activity. Increasing the level of "free" or usable catecholamines in rats by administering an antidepressant drug produces negative effects on the reproductive cycle, including prevention of implantation of fertilized eggs into the uterine wall, interruption of estrus (fertility) cycles, delayed onset of estrus in young mice, and lowering of the weight of reproductive organs in young mice.[7]

Progesterone may serve as some protection against the potentially harmful effects of excess catecholamines. Some of the effects produced in the rodent studies were partially reversible with the administration of progesterone. Rodent studies also suggest an inverse relationship between norepinephrine and progesterone; levels of the former are at their lowest when progesterone is at its peak. Consistent with these findings, it is now established that progesterone increases the levels of the chemical *monoamine oxidase* (MAO), which is most responsible for the breakdown and deactivation of norepinephrine. The connection between norepinephrine and progesterone is worth considering in a discussion of the psychology of the pregnant woman, since a well-known hypothesis holds that many depressions may be associated with norepinephrine deficiency. One study did indeed find evidence of a deficiency of usable norepinephrine in pregnant subjects with emotional changes including decreased interest in social activities, a decreased startle response, and increased depression.[8] Although recent research questions the exact relationship of norepinephrine deficiency to depression, no one doubts that this essential neurotransmitter plays a role in the biology of emotion.

The demonstrated relationship of progesterone to the action of norepinephrine is just one example of how this steroid has been associated with physical changes that might produce depression. Evidence is strong that progesterone has a sedative effect on the central nervous system. For example, EEGs of pregnant women show slowing of brain waves. In animal studies, the administration of progesterone produces general anesthesia, especially in females. In humans, researchers have been able to induce sleep by administering progesterone intravenously. A study of epileptic women showed fewer seizures when progesterone is high in the latter half of the menstrual cycle and increased seizure activity when progesterone is lowest (around the time of the menstrual period). When these subjects received premenstrual doses of progesterone, seizure activity decreased.[9] Finally, in some animals, progesterone changes the arousal threshold; that is, greater stimulus is needed to produce a reaction.[10] This finding is consistent with the decreased startle response noted in pregnant women. In all, there is clear evidence that pregnancy causes a change in a woman's reactivity.

The change in reactivity could well be a protective measure for the fetus. By inhibiting smooth muscle activity, progesterone may prevent premature uterine contractions. One woman interviewed for this book who did experience premature contractions reported that they were brought on by the slightest emotional stress—even watching a scary movie on television. This woman's experience demonstrates how emotional reactions and muscular activity can be related and why reduced reactivity may benefit the fetus.

Unfortunately, for some mothers the effect of these hormonal mediations may be less salutary than it is for the fetus. Pregnant women have complained of "fogginess" and have shown poor performance (compared to nonpregnant subjects) on cognitive tests. (Similarly, some oral contraceptive users have complained of feeling less responsive to the environment.) For some pregnant women, these feelings may become more pronounced and eventually develop into clinical depression.

One measure of the body's reactivity is the release of cortisol, a steroid that, like the catecholamines, is produced when the body requires arousal. Like progesterone, cortisol is present in unusual amounts in pregnancy, with concentrations rising threefold over nonpregnant levels by late pregnancy. In a nonpregnant person, such concentrations would almost certainly produce signs of hypercortisolism (most often seen in patients receiving high or continuous doses of corticosteroids such as some anti-asthma medications). However, these signs, such as a round "moon" face and skin that is easily bruised, are not normally present in pregnant women despite the exaggerated cortisol levels.

It may be that high levels of progesterone mediate against such effects in pregnant women. In order to be transported through the blood, cortisol has to bind itself to certain protein molecules. Progesterone inhibits the activity of cortisol to some degree by occupying the binding sites on those molecules. Imagine cortisol and progesterone, both in high concentrations during pregnancy, going head-to-head in your pregnant body, competing for important binding sites like Christmas shoppers fighting for parking spaces. Is it possible that your mood is somewhat dependent on which shoppers hold the upper hand?

Measurement of cortisol reactivity—that is, how cortisol levels changed in response to stress—was the basis of a study of pregnant adolescents that attempted to associate stress with depression. The hypothesis was that subjects with increased cortisol reactivity would be more anxious and depressed during pregnancy. The researchers did find a significant connection between cortisol reactivity and depression, but not the connection they expected. Instead, they found that subjects with increased reactivity showed less depression. A *decrease* in reactivity turned out to be a reliable predictor of depression in early pregnancy.[11]

Perhaps this finding surprised the researchers, but it makes sense in the context of human behavior under stress. When stressful circumstances arise, the people who cope best are those able to react. Even reactions that may not seem like positive adaptations afford some feeling of control. It seems likely that a pregnant woman who feels unable to react to her new situation will suffer some degree of depression, especially in our modern world, where many women are accustomed to being in control of their circumstances.

Other studies have confirmed a reduced reactivity in pregnancy in other ways. One study showed that test situations designed to elicit elevations in blood pressure have a reduced effect in pregnant women, whose blood vessels simply fail to rise to the challenge.[12] In fact, the lowered blood pressure of normal pregnancy may in itself predispose women to depressive symptoms. In some studies of nonpregnant subjects low blood pressure has been associated with tiredness, dizziness, headache, anxiety, depression, fatigue, and a readiness to cry.[13]

In the end, however, the greatest part of pregnancy depression likely boils down to the obvious culprit: hormones. It's a word you will hear too often in these nine long months, but given the undeniable and complex connections between hormones and mood, coupled with the dramatic changes in the levels and metabolism of hormones in pregnancy, it seems impossible to overstress their role in how you or any other pregnant woman feels from day to day.

Remember, though, that these hormones are not playing their roles inside a test tube, but inside a body—a body with a history, surrounded by an environment. In the delicate chemistry of brain and emotion, biology cannot act independently of psychosocial influences, including everything from early childhood experiences to current circumstances. This combination makes it hard to sort out emotions in pregnancy, as Barbara, who had suffered some depressive episodes before pregnancy, recalled:

> I started seeing a therapist in the middle of the second trimester of my second pregnancy. I went and saw a woman, a social worker somebody had recommended, and she was like, "So you're feeling *bad*." And I'm like, "Yes, I'm feeling *bad*, that's why I'm here." And I knew it was something deeper than that, that I had to go back and pick up the work I'd started in previous therapy. So we got in touch with this therapist. . . . But the whole time I was there, I remember saying, "I feel *this*, and I feel *this*, but I don't know whether it's because I'm just pregnant." I really had a hard time differentiating between what was old issues and what was hormone-induced.

> I didn't know if I needed to just kind of relax and go with it, just say, "I'm not going to act on this; I'm not going to try to fix it." But the fear of ever falling back into that same old depression said, "No, I'm going to keep going to somebody."

Barbara undoubtedly made an appropriate choice—not because her depression was not a biological phenomenon, but because that phenomenon was occurring in the presence of both old and new issues that required confrontation. As far as anyone has been able to relate life events to depression, pregnancy meets every criterion for the kind of event virtually guaranteed to bring on psychological earthquakes. There is no escaping the stressors of such a life-changing event, but many factors, from genetic makeup to learning to environmental influences, may determine how those stressors affect each woman. Taken together, these factors constitute an individual's *vulnerability* to depression.

Maybe your first exposure to the concept of vulnerability came with Superman, who was *invulnerable*. Nothing could hurt him—not bullets, not falling buildings, not lack of intimacy with Lois Lane. However, for mere mortals, vulnerability is part of the psychological and physical makeup. Part of that vulnerability is genetically determined. Another part is probably learned and consists of a series of habitual reactions to stressors. These habits are acquired over the course of a lifetime but are heavily influenced by the circumstances of your early years. Evidence now accumulating suggests that the pathways over which neurotransmitters interact are shaped according to whether an individual successfully adapts or fails to adapt to stressful changes.[14] Thus the influences of your childhood, your learned patterns of response to stressful events, could biologically predispose you to depressive symptoms when pregnancy disarranges the interactions of your neurotransmitters.

Also important are the social circumstances surrounding a stressful event. Given the widely differing circumstances of individual lives, there is no reason why the same event should carry the same meaning or produce the same reaction in any two people. Among the *vulnerability factors*, things that make you more liable to hurt, that have been postulated are lack of an intimate companion, responsibility for the care of young children, and the lack of a social support network. While these are not proven risk factors for depressive illness, any or all may figure into the life of a pregnant woman, influencing her mental state to some degree. Jae described how the circumstances surrounding a pregnancy influenced her feelings:

> I was really depressed at the end of my first pregnancy. I don't know how much of that was circumstances of my life at the time

> and how much was hormones of being pregnant. We had just moved and so I lost all of my friends, my support group, my church, all the women I was pregnant with (I had a bunch of friends who were all pregnant at the same time). Didn't know anybody, didn't have anything to do. I was bored silly! And I was used to working 60 hours a week . . . and all of a sudden I had nothing to do with my time. And I'm very much a doer. So that was really frustrating for me. And my expectations at the time were that we were going to set everything up and make it look pretty, and get my nursery ready for my baby—and our apartment was not finished, and it ended up being finished the day before I gave birth! So that was very stressful for me.

With a melee of conflicting studies, psychiatrists have sought some way of predicting which life events will place stress on most individuals. In an attempt to evaluate the stressfulness of events with some consistency, they have focused on two measures: the undesirability of an event and the amount of change that event will produce in the life of the individual. As an event that may score high in the first category (depending on the woman's circumstances) and goes way over the top in the second, pregnancy certainly ranks high as a stressful experience.

In fact, psychologists call pregnancy a *developmental crisis*, meaning that it involves mental and physical changes so profound as to constitute a point of no return. The pregnant woman must define a new role for herself and move forward into it, which calls for a series of adjustments involving tremendous mental strain. Most psychological profiles of pregnancy describe it as a time when previously repressed feelings come to the surface and clamor for attention. Most of these are highly charged emotional issues. (If they weren't, they wouldn't have been repressed in the first place.) Sexuality naturally figures into the process, as do a woman's feelings about and relationship with her own mother. These specters haunt the sub-basements and crawl spaces of any woman's personality, and when they suddenly appear on the ground floor, virtually no woman escapes the encounter unshaken.

In societies where magic and superstition play an acknowledged role in daily life, the powerful emotional aspects of pregnancy are recognized with rituals and taboos. So-called developed societies have their own rituals, such as baby showers, as well as taboos against certain foods or activities. Also common worldwide, apparently, is the pregnant woman's tending to become the property of the community. (How many strangers ever patted you on the abdomen *before* you became pregnant?) A study on pregnancy and mental health in rural Africa notes that "all human communities regard the pregnant woman as a special person and expect the woman (as she does herself) to feel normal and happy in her condition."[15] Unfortunately for this pregnant woman, both the mental and the physical attributes of her condition may predispose her not to happiness but to uncertainty and depression. Knowing that she is expected to be glowing with happiness when she actually feels terrible can only make the depression worse. She judges herself, as Barbara did:

> To complicate matters, while I was having an "I'm depressed" feeling, my ego or superego or whatever was judging the feelings I was having: "You *ought* to be grateful. You *ought* to feel good. You *know* what a joy having a child is; you already have one. . . ." And yet there was a child screaming in there that said, "This isn't fair, I don't like it, I'm uncomfortable, I'm sad, I'm miserable!"

There is that child in all of us—plus the whole of our adult lives, plus the biology that brought us from childhood to adulthood to pregnancy. Each of these things influences how we function, so that in the end, pinpointing one biological or psychosocial factor as the source of all depressive symptoms is no more correct than writing it off as a bad attitude. It is clear that the experience of depressive symptoms involves a lengthy chain of complex interactions along pathways that may have been formed by events in the distant past. No two women, therefore, are likely to experience depression or anything else about pregnancy in exactly the same way. At the same time, accumulating evidence suggests that depressive symptoms are both common and explicable in pregnancy. No woman need ever feel that she suffers alone.

We are all vulnerable to some degree, and perhaps never more so than when we open ourselves to the attachment of a new human being. The decision to bear a child is not always recognized as the act of bravery it really is. If your circumstances—whether genetic, biochemical, environmental, or psychosocial—have left you especially vulnerable to physical and emotional stress, you are the more to be commended for your willingness to take on the demands of pregnancy. To those who take the greatest risks come the greatest rewards, and your rewards are waiting just ahead.

Feeling Better

Lack of attention to or understanding of subclinical depression has perhaps resulted in a lack of appropriate treatment. Around the 1960s, it became the common practice for physicians to jump on a woman's depressive symptoms with both feet (and with prescription pads in both hands), and some of the literature from those years suggests that some physicians were likely too quick to interpret mood changes in pregnancy as depressive illness requiring treatment. In 1961, one physician wrote that he had studied fifty-five pregnant women and determined that forty-seven of them required medication for depressive states. Three of these subjects found that the medication–the amphetamine desoxyephedrine–gave them more energy than they could handle; to these three, the doctor also prescribed a sedative, sodium pentobarbital, to be taken in combination with the amphetamine. The other forty-four patients took daily doses of desoxyephedrine ranging from 5 to 15 milligrams. Of the twenty-two taking the highest dose, nine took an additional dose eight to ten hours later. (Most of this last group "had a multitude of household duties requiring sixteen or more hours per day of physical effort," which could go a long way toward explaining their depressive states). Though each woman discontinued the study doses after the sixteenth week of pregnancy, each was allowed to continue the medication by choice. After intervals of three to twenty-three days without medication, thirty-four of the forty-seven patients began taking the amphetamine again "because they appreciated the increased sense of energy and drive."[16]

Today this picture conjures up some pretty horrifying parallels for anyone who has ever fed pleasure pills to rats in a college psychology experiment, and one hopes that physicians have become more conservative about what kind of drugs they prescribe to pregnant women and in what amounts. One also hopes that the modern obstetrician understands enough about the biological and psychosocial facets of depression not to write off a pregnant woman's symptoms as "dread . . . of the extended physical changes incongruous with the latest clothes and footwear."[17]

However, the treatments most frequently prescribed for depressive symptoms are still treatments for full-fledged depression–psychotherapy or antidepressant medication. For the type of subclinical depression most women experience in pregnancy, these treatments may prove inappropriately lengthy and needlessly expensive (psychotherapy is both the longest and, in some cases, the costliest form of treatment), ineffective (antidepressants have apparently not been proved effective for mild mood disturbances), or even dangerous (psychotherapeutic drugs are generally not recommended for use in pregnancy). In some cases, simply attending a support group may be more effective and appropriate than any of these treatments.[18] Your county department of social services (usually listed in the phone book with other county offices) can steer you toward such support groups or other helpful services in your area.

On the other hand, some of the nonpharmacological treatments currently used for clinical depression might prove very beneficial in pregnancy were anyone to test them. The following therapies are directed toward mechanisms that have a lot in common with the circumstances of pregnancy.

Bright light therapy. Intriguing similarities exist between the depressive pattern of early pregnancy and seasonal affective disorder, a depressive illness whose symptoms occur only in the fall and winter. The symptoms, which include not only sadness and irritability but cravings for carbohydrates, daytime drowsiness and excessive sleeping, lack of energy, and difficulty concentrating or interacting with others at home or on the job, probably sound familiar to many pregnant women. Even more striking, however, is the connection that pregnancy-related and seasonal depression may share between symptoms and the release of the hormone *melatonin*.

Like many hormones, melatonin is synthesized and released in a twenty-four-hour rhythm. Normally (in persons not working the night shift), the production of melatonin is related to darkness; the highest levels of melatonin in the blood occur between midnight and 6:00 A.M. Researchers have found that bright light suppresses melatonin release and that continued suppression relieves the symptoms of seasonal affective disorder. Conversely, dosing patients with melatonin reduces the therapeutic effect of light. Melatonin, then, has a clear influence on the symptoms of seasonal affective disorder.

A study of sleep disturbance in pregnancy found that pregnant subjects showed higher levels of melatonin than nonpregnant women. The study authors suggest that bright light therapy may alleviate sleep problems for some pregnant women.[19] Bright light has already proved beneficial in the treatment of a patient with premenstrual symptoms that showed a seasonal pattern.[20] It seems quite possible that pregnant women with depressive symptoms could also benefit from a course of phototherapy.

Bright light therapy involves a daily period (usually one to two hours) of sitting in front of a specially constructed light box designed to provide light about five times brighter than standard office lighting. The timing of this period is important and must be determined by the therapist. (If the therapy seems ineffective, a change in session timing could make a difference.) General recommendations indicate that patients may read or work in front of the box so long as they remember to glance up at the lights a few times per minute. Results may be evident in as little as four days, and the course of therapy is short overall, perhaps two weeks.[21]

It has been suggested that seasonal affective disorder may be something like a hibernation response in humans.[22] If you feel that pregnancy is driving you underground for a long cold spell, bright light therapy may be a promising option for you. It is certainly worth discussing with your heath care provider.

Exercise. Whether you have been pregnant long enough to read only one other pregnancy book or twelve others, you have been urged to exercise. Moderate, regular exercise in pregnancy has been credited with benefits ranging from improving overall fitness to increasing energy, reducing constipation, and alleviating headache. Another likely benefit is improved mood. Many studies have demonstrated that among the population at large, exercise helps to relieve depressive symptoms and establish a feeling of well-being. Significantly, these studies are not examining the "runner's high" that got a lot of press during the craze for distance running (the endorphin rush of the athlete pushing beyond normal endurance). Instead, findings suggest that comfortable levels of activity are sufficient to maintain improved mood. Doctors prescribe walking, swimming, bicycling, or aerobic dance to combat depression. Nonaerobic exercise such as weight lifting may be equally effective in relieving depressive symptoms.[23] (See Appendix for further discussion of exercise in pregnancy.)

For a long time, the mood-improving effects of exercise were trivialized by the assumption that having physically conditioned, better-looking bodies simply made people feel better about themselves. However, studies have found that subjects do not need to attain aerobic fitness or lose any weight to enjoy relief from depression through exercise. The assumption that improved appearance is all it takes to relieve depression is about on par with the idea that depression in pregnancy is caused solely by concern about weight gain. There is more to depression, and likely more to exercise, than that.

Indeed, it seems likely that like depression itself, the benefits of exercise in relieving depression arise from the fundamental chemistry of brain and personality. Exercise alters levels of neurotransmitters. If regular exercise helps to sustain high levels of serotonin, as studies suggest, the increased stability of the serotonergic system may help combat mood disturbance. Catecholamine levels, too, increase with exercise and may likewise serve to stabilize neurotransmission and lift the spirits.

Exercise is cheap or free, beneficial in many respects for you and your developing child, carries no warning labels (apart from the caution of moderation in pregnancy), and is available everywhere. Avail yourself of its many benefits, and your spirits may reward you.

Vitamin B_6 (pyridoxine). As mentioned earlier, some researchers have suggested that depression associated with the use of oral contraceptives may be related to a steroid-induced deficiency of vitamin B_6. That deficiency interferes with the conversion of the amino acid tryptophan to the neurotransmitter serotonin. Accordingly, some doctors have recommended B_6 supplements as a therapy for depression. In one study, two doctors in Wisconsin prescribed doses of 50 milligrams per day for patients with depression related to oral contraceptive use. Forty-four out of fifty-eight patients experienced either complete relief or considerable improvement of their depressive symptoms. Three pregnant patients who also took B_6 for depression enjoyed similar results.[24]

The findings of this study suggest that when B_6 works, it works very well. Subjects who experienced improvement noticed results within twenty-four hours. A woman who increased her dosage to 100 milligrams per day was rewarded with too much energy and difficulty sleeping. However, for the fourteen patients who experienced no improvement with B_6, doubling the dosage had no effect. These findings seem to confirm that no therapy will work the same way for everyone—not surprising, considering the complex and individual chain of events that constitutes depression. All the same, anything that has helped even one other pregnant woman is probably worth considering.

However, do not supplement with B_6, or any vitamin, without discussing it with your doctor. There is a popular notion that a water-soluble vitamin cannot reach toxic levels in the body, but at least in the case of B_6, research suggests otherwise. There have been several reported cases of people who temporarily lost their ability to walk or balance or suffered other signs of central nervous system disorder from overdoses of B_6. Granted, the doses required to produce these signs of toxicity were huge—2 grams or more a day (a typical prenatal vitamin contains only 10 milligrams) for long periods. Nevertheless, the central nervous system of mammals appears to be vulnerable to harm from overdoses of B_6.[25] Be sure to take into consideration all sources of B_6—diet, prenatal vitamins, and supplements—when discussing dosage with your doctor.

Sleep deprivation. This therapy for depression is new, largely untried, unexplained, and evidently not for everyone. In fact, to an exhausted pregnant woman, it may be the most unappealing treatment ever suggested. Nevertheless, a recent work on depression claims that staying awake all night has offered temporary relief of depression to some patients.[26] No one knows how it works, but if your college experience included the giddiness that tends to follow an all-night study session, you can imagine that this cure might have sprung from the addled brain of a medical intern on a thirty-six-hour shift. At any rate, the recent text emphasizes that sleep deprivation is an experimental therapy that patients should not attempt to practice on themselves unsupervised. If you are interested in this treatment, you should consult a health practitioner with experience in its use—who, considering the experimental nature of the therapy, may be extremely difficult to find. It wouldn't hurt, though, to start with your own doctor, who not only knows how to research it but has also graduated from medical school and has therefore had at least some experience with pulling all-nighters.

Some Thoughts on Medication

When depressive symptoms appear for the first time in pregnancy, a physician today is likely to take a cautious and conservative approach toward therapy. Weighing the largely unknown risks of psychoactive drugs to the fetus against the probability that depression will improve by the second trimester, a physician probably will prefer to explore other treatment options—and there is much that a supportive, sympathetic practitioner can do to help simply by being willing to consider the problem seriously.

Nevertheless, a substantial number of women do take psychoactive drugs at some point in their pregnancies. Often women are using the medication when they conceive, so the question is not whether to begin antidepressant medication in pregnancy but whether to stop.

There is no way to prove that a medication will not harm a fetus. Even massive clinical trials could not assure 100 percent safety—and massive clinical trials are not conducted on pregnant women. After all, a drug manufacturer can't ask large numbers of pregnant women to ingest an experimental drug in order to determine its effects. For this reason, shocking though it may seem, most drugs win FDA approval for marketing with no investigation of their effect on human fetuses.

Reports on the potentially harmful effects of a drug are limited mostly to two sources: anecdotal reports of pregnancies that occurred while women were taking the drug and animal studies. Both sources are, to say the least, unreliable. What happens to a drug inside a sheep or rat or monkey may not happen inside a human. (The unreliability of animal data was amply demonstrated in the 1950s when Thalidomide, which showed no harmful effects in animal fetuses, left many children across Europe with major limb deformities.) Anecdotal reports of human pregnancies are sometimes more helpful, particularly when they show a rare birth defect occurring in numbers of infants. However, a collection of these reports is not the same thing as a controlled clinical study, and the data may be skewed by genetic, environmental, or other factors.

Because drugs are not tested on pregnant women before marketing, data on potential risks to fetuses begin to accumulate only after a drug hits the shelves. For this reason, it is often the case that the newer the drug, the scantier the information on its effects in pregnancy. This presents problems for women taking perhaps the most popular antidepressant, Prozac (fluoxetine), approved for the market in 1987. However, the popularity of the drug provides a sample base even at this early stage.

A 1991 report from Prozac's manufacturer, Eli Lilly, covers 219 pregnancies. Of these, 128 births were considered normal. Thirty-nine pregnancies were terminated by elective abortion. The number of miscarriages (twenty-nine pregnancies) was slightly higher than the normal incidence in the population at large. There were ten premature births. There were major malformations in six births, but because there were no similarities among these, it is not possible to associate any of them with the use of Prozac.[27]

Antidepressants such as imipramine, desipramine, and amitriptyline have been in use much longer, but available data are not much more revealing. Research has established that imipramine and desipramine readily cross the placenta, but beyond that studies are inconclusive, despite the larger number of reports available. Some reports suggest a link between imipramine and desipramine and fetal limb malformations, but other sources, including a study of more than 2,700 births, have failed to confirm the association.[28]

The case against lithium, the drug most commonly prescribed for manic-depressive (bipolar) disorder, is much stronger. Since 1968 there has been a central source, the International Register of Lithium Babies, for recording the outcomes of births to mothers who took lithium at any time during pregnancy. Evidence increasingly suggests that lithium taken in the first trimester produces birth defects in humans, especially defects of the cardiovascular system. Among the defects recorded by the Register are six cases of an extremely rare heart defect called Ebstein's anomaly. That six such cases should appear among only 225 births is almost irrefutable evidence that lithium use was involved. There are also dangers involved with taking the drug later in pregnancy, especially at term, since newborn infants exposed to lithium just before birth have displayed many problems, including flaccid muscle tone, poor sucking reflexes, and lethargy.[29]

What are the risks of abstaining from medication for depression or other mental disorders during pregnancy? For women with a history of suicide fantasies or attempts, the mother's life may be in danger. In such cases the physician may well decide that untreated depression poses more of a risk than medication for both mother and child. However, many other women find that the risk of depression does not have to be life-threatening to be terrifying.

Barbara describes the feelings that shaped her decision to continue Prozac in her first pregnancy:

> Prior to my getting pregnant with my first child, the depressions had been severe. . . . It wasn't a suicidal thing, but if somebody had run over me, that wouldn't have been a problem with me. I felt like if I carried a child and was as depressed as I had been, then that wouldn't be any better than some unknown risk of some pharmaceutical. The known, the bleakness of depression, to me outweighed that risk.

Deciding what to do about medication during pregnancy may be one of the hardest decisions you'll ever make, and you should not do it alone. Read everything you can find. Explore the issue with your doctor, your partner, and anyone else who can give you support and advice. In these explorations, however, do not allow anyone to trivialize the challenge you face. Pregnancy is short only to those not experiencing it, and the uninitiated cannot possibly understand what it means to give over the control of your body to another human life. Not everyone can relinquish that control, knowing what may lie on the other side of surrender. Be true to yourself, and make the best, most informed decision you can. A world of women is standing behind you.

4

Fatigue

If the training of your health care provider included standard obstetrical texts, he or she has ingested the following remarks on fatigue in pregnancy: (1) It is very common in the first trimester; (2) it usually goes away by the fourth month; and (3) it has (according to *Williams Obstetrics*) "no special significance."[1]

As with many other pregnancy complaints, a discussion of fatigue raises questions about medical versus personal "significance." As a measure of your health or the progress of your pregnancy, fatigue does not suggest any problem and is therefore not medically significant. On the other hand, what is the significance of fatigue in the life of a pregnant woman?

"I was a full-time student during my first trimester of pregnancy," wrote Linda Sue. "I was so fatigued I had to cut back to part-time." Writing at 31 weeks, Linda noted that the fatigue "is back now, as bad" as in the early weeks.

Colleen, describing a first trimester marred by extreme emotional problems and exhaustion, said:

> I was so tired. I was helping my boyfriend's mother building miniature dollhouses, and doing these little things. I would sit there and just feel totally exhausted as soon as I got there, and she just told me to go home. But I had a hard time sleeping, even though I was just exhausted all the time.

Said Kim S.:

> I think that it's hard for employers to understand just how exhausted you are and how difficult it is. Before I knew that I was pregnant, one of the things that clued me in was that two Saturdays in a row, I literally slept all day. And I was thinking, What is

> going on? I am so exhausted! I would come home after a week of teaching, and I would sleep all day long. Fortunately, during my pregnancy my work situation was good in that I was teaching special extension and had a wonderful teaching assistant who had already had two children. She would look at me and say, "You just go in the back room and lie down on the couch." And I would often do that, probably two or three times a day. So I was in a work environment where I had some support. But I never actually told my boss that I was lying down three times a day!

Because fatigue does not appear to affect or predict the outcome of pregnancy, research on the symptom is scarce indeed. However, in recent years the problem has begun to receive attention in the literature of nursing and midwifery. Research so far, though still extremely scanty and based on small samples, has offered important insights into the incidence of fatigue in pregnancy and its relationship to other factors.

Were you not already collapsed on the couch, the incidence figures would stagger you: In early pregnancy, about 90 percent of women report feelings of fatigue. (Thus your OB's training is evidently on target here, though for "very common" you might wish to substitute "practically inescapable.") Research suggests, however, that despite the textbook view, the symptom does not disappear at the end of the first trimester. In one study, 100 percent of subjects complained of fatigue in late pregnancy.[2]

Why are pregnant women so exhausted? To begin with the obvious culprits, consider the dramatic changes pregnancy forces on the body. First of all, your fetus is not the only one growing. You are going through a period of rapid cell proliferation, developing new muscles in the uterus, sprouting glandular tissue in the breasts, and spinning a tremendous network of new blood vessels. In a nonpregnant adult, such sudden and rapid growth signifies serious disease, which certainly suggests that your body might be highly stressed by the activity. Furthermore, structures that are not growing are working harder than usual. By the end of the first trimester, your heart is pumping out from 20 to 50 percent more blood and doing it faster (ten to fifteen more beats per minute). Your lungs are holding more air. Some 25 to 50 percent more blood is flowing through your kidneys, expecting to be filtered. All these changes are accompanied by a significant increase in your overall metabolism, reflected by a rise in your basal body temperature, which stays elevated until midpregnancy. Finally, to support all this activity, your body consumes 14 to 20 percent more oxygen than normal. These factors in combination result in tremendous energy depletion, placing the exhaustion most women feel in pregnancy squarely within the definition of fatigue as a "state of increased discomfort and decreased efficiency resulting from expenditure of energy reserve."[3]

Yet the experience of fatigue is more complex, involving one's perceptions of self and of how that self performs in an accustomed environment. These perceptions are affected by various physical, psychological, and environmental factors. One team of researchers,[4] apparently the first to undertake a study specifically researching the problem of fatigue in pregnancy, worked within a model of fatigue that considered many variables, including the subject's state of physical conditioning (energy potential), sleep patterns, other disease states, self-confidence in performing physical tasks, motivation to perform tasks, amount and intensity of physical and mental work to be accomplished, and environmental factors such as the season of the year (which might involve changes in temperature, humidity, or allergens). As these researchers noted, even assuming that fatigue is stimulated by the physical changes of pregnancy, any of the variables in their model might contribute to the severity and duration of that fatigue.

The results of this study showed correlations between certain variables and the severity of fatigue. According to these results, age may make a difference, though not in the way you might expect: Younger women tended to have higher fatigue scores. Unsurprisingly, greater fatigue tended to accompany greater nausea. High fatigue scores also showed up in women who gained less weight in pregnancy—an intriguing finding because it seems to counter the assumption that fatigue in pregnancy is related to the effort of carrying excess weight. Perhaps the lower weight gain occurred in the more nauseated (and thus more fatigued) group; or perhaps lower weight gain and fatigue both indicated energy expenditure even greater than the level expected in pregnancy.

A surprising finding was that amount of sleep did not appear to correlate with feelings of fatigue. Many women in the study cited extra sleep as their main mechanism for coping with fatigue, yet the scores do not suggest that these women felt any less tired than those who did not get extra sleep. Furthermore, many study subjects reported feeling tired even upon awakening from sleep, as Dawn T. described: "During the second and third month, I would fall asleep about 7:00 P.M., get up at 7:00 A.M., and still be tired."

Also surprising was that fatigue was apparently independent of such variables as number of children and number of hours worked outside the home. Naturally, one would expect that caring for other children or working outside the home (or, especially, both) would add to a woman's exhaustion, but in fact the women not shouldering these burdens were not relieved of fatigue. All in all, pregnant women just plain felt tired, no matter how frantic or peaceful their lives and no matter how many hours they clocked in bed.

The findings of this study cannot be taken as gospel. For one thing, the study included only thirty subjects, and the results may be skewed by certain selection factors. However, the authors draw on their results to make an important observation: If fatigue in pregnancy is indeed so little related to external factors such as workload and so little relieved by rest, the symptom is likely produced or influenced by hormonal factors apart from the energy-draining effects of mechanical body changes.

As possible support for this hypothesis, the authors cite an apparent relationship between fatigue and mood states. Women with high fatigue scores also tended to report more feelings of anxiety, anger, depression, and confusion. Women who reported feeling tired upon awakening were also more likely to report anger, depression, and confusion. It seems clear that fatigue and mood states are related, but is it sufficient to explain the connection by pointing out that being tired makes you crabby? If it were a simple cause-and-effect relationship, why would the fatigue and the mood states not be relieved by rest? Instead, it seems quite possible that the same (probably hormonal) influences that cause the fatigue are also affecting the emotions.

Altogether, it seems that the popular image of the energetic pregnant woman, slashing and burning her way through her household chores in a nesting fever, is considerably at odds with the way most women experience pregnancy. Seventy percent of study subjects indicated that fatigue had forced them to adjust their schedules at home, reducing housework and social activity in favor of napping or going to bed earlier at night. Even so, only 36 percent stated that fatigue had increased their dependence on others—spouse, housekeeper/baby-sitter, or children—for household management.[5] Perhaps the latter finding hints at an exacerbating factor of pregnancy fatigue: the pregnant woman's determination to shoulder her burdens alone.

Suppose you decide to take a nap at a time when you'd usually be cleaning up after a meal. If you have not "increased your dependence" to the point of asking for a little help with the dishes, you are not likely to feel rested upon awakening, since the first thing you'll see is the dishes still sitting on the kitchen table. Whatever the hormonal or mechanical causes of fatigue, it is no surprise that extra sleep should fail to relieve exhaustion when the sleep results in a pile of neglected chores topped by a large load of guilt. Unfortunately, it is likely that many women find themselves in this fatigue-perpetuating cycle because they feel pressured to preserve an illusion of perfect strength—an illusion that includes no accommodation for the workings of the female body.

Such pressure is even more evident in the study findings about fatigue and employment. Out of thirty subjects, only three responded that fatigue had caused them to adjust their activities at work. All three of these reported that their adjustment strategy was to reduce their hours.[6] Perhaps it was easier simply not to be at work (and live on a reduced income) than to risk less vigorous performance on the job.

We begin to see (obstetrical texts please take note) how fatigue assumes significance in the life of a pregnant woman. First, it is apparent that many pregnant women feel tremendous pressure *not to be tired.* Since this pressure is often strongest on the job, women exert unusual effort to maintain the illusion of energy during working hours. The resulting backlash fatigue often proves disruptive to home and family. If pressures in the home drive a woman to continue that schedule uninterrupted, disruptions may be turned entirely inward, placing body and soul at risk of harm.

Feeling Better

Fatigue is a protective symptom, a warning that the body's energy is depleted, significantly reducing its ability to cope with stressors.[7] Therapies therefore attempt to build up that ability. None of these therapies has been studied on a wide scale for use in pregnancy, and success rates are mixed. However, none is harmful, and each has helped some woman in some way.

Relaxation. Don't just rest–*relax.* Relaxation is not vegging out in front of the television, but a series of learned responses based on a knowledge of the muscular system. It is the foundation of yoga, transcendental meditation, and biofeedback–all of which are accessible to you through local classes, medical centers, or private teachers. If consciously and conscientiously pursued, relaxation offers great benefits. It has been shown to decrease oxygen consumption (proposed as a factor in pregnancy fatigue) more than sleep does. Herbert Benson, in his book *The Relaxation Response,* noted that while sleep decreased oxygen consumption 8 percent over a period of four to five hours, relaxation exercises produced a decrease of 10 to 20 percent in three minutes. These impressive findings suggest that relaxation exercises, performed during short breaks throughout the workday, may go a long way toward relieving the fatigue of a pregnant woman in the workplace, where afternoon naps are probably not possible.[8]

Exercise. Aerobic and muscle-strengthening exercises may also help combat fatigue. Swimming and brisk walking are two of the finest aerobic exercises a pregnant woman can enjoy. (See other exercise guidelines in the Appendix.) A study of exercise in pregnancy found that pregnant women who participated in moderate aerobic exercise reported less fatigue than their non-exercising counterparts (as well as fewer backaches, headaches, and hot flashes and less shortness of breath). The authors speculate that reduced tension, increased self-esteem and improved muscle tone, all proven results of exercise, may be responsible for the decrease in fatigue.[9] Also important are specific muscle-tightening exercises, which can reduce fatiguing strain on the back, abdomen, and pelvic muscles without taxing the body's already depleted energy resources. Many such exercises can be incorporated into daily routines: contracting and releasing the abdominal muscles while waiting in line, tightening these muscles and squatting to lift objects, stretching the legs and ankles with ankle rotations when feet are elevated, or performing Kegel exercises (see Chapter 14) at "cue" times throughout the day (waiting at red lights, washing the dishes).[10]

Then again, exercise may not prove much of a remedy if you are already running yourself ragged. "I was tired a lot during my second pregnancy because my first was still so young," said Diane. "They're seventeen months apart. It was so much work because he was so active, so it was just running around and running around. I was trying to exercise at the same time and then I finally gave that up." Or, as Ann wrote more succinctly, "Forget an exercise routine. All I wanted was sleep (and food)!"

Dietary remedies. Food, actually, is a fine remedy in itself. Remember that your body's normal signals may be disrupted, and hunger may deplete your energy before you even feel your stomach is empty. The standard advice applies: Eat snacks high in protein and carbohydrate but low in sugar to avoid even worse fatigue from dramatic swings in blood sugar.

Vitamins are also important. One nutritional remedy long recommended for relief of fatigue is vitamin B_6 (pyridoxine). Two doctors in Wisconsin conducted a study on the efficacy of B_6 in relieving certain symptoms associated with the use of oral contraceptives, fatigue among them (along with depression, mood swings, difficulty concentrating, sleep disturbance, and mild feelings of paranoia).[11] These doctors pointed to evidence suggesting that depression with oral contraceptive use might be due in part to the interaction of the pill with vitamin B_6. Estrogens may interfere with the body's ability to use B_6 efficiently, creating a so-called functional deficiency (that is, the vitamin is present but not being used). That deficiency, in turn, may cause a disruption of the normal conversion of the amino acid tryptophan to the neurotransmitter serotonin, and disturbed serotonin levels are believed to be responsible for some symptoms of depression.

When subjects in the Wisconsin study ingested 50 milligrams of B_6 a day, a majority found their symptoms, including fatigue, either completely relieved or considerably improved within twenty-four hours. (One woman found 50 milligrams so satisfactory that she decided on her own to increase her dose to 100 milligrams a day, at which point she began experiencing excess energy and disturbed sleep patterns and was forced to reduce the dose.) Because pregnancy produces a similar disturbance of the tryptophan metabolism, these doctors also included a few pregnant women in their study, with similar good results.

It is worth noting, however, that the fourteen (of fifty-eight) subjects who showed no improvement with 50 milligrams experienced no greater success with 100 milligrams. Even if the vitamin works as well as this study seems to demonstrate, its effects are apparently not universal, which suggests that both cause and cure of fatigue and depression are inextricably entwined with individual biology.

Do not supplement with B_6 without discussing it with your doctor. There do appear to be hazards associated with its overuse.[12] Although the doses that have produced problems (such as difficulty walking or loss of balance) have been enormous—at least 2 grams a day for extended periods—the reported cases have all been nonpregnant adults. There are no reports of how large doses of B_6 might affect a developing fetus. Be sure to consider all your sources of B_6, including diet, when consulting with your doctor about supplementation.

Because pregnancy is a continuously stressful state, you may feel some fatigue throughout. But while you may not be able to eliminate fatigue altogether, you can set two goals. First, keep it from disrupting your personal life. Talk openly with family, coworkers, and anyone else whose understanding is important to your well-being. Linda Sue, who said her fatigue and irritability "strained the relationship with my eighteen-year-old stepson," enlisted the help of her husband, who "took over most of the contact with him and explained the situation to him. By the time my stepson moved out, our relationship was better from having shared with him honestly the changes I was going through. (Maybe he'll be more supportive of his future wife!)" When fatigue forced Linda Sue to cut back on her hours as a student, she explained her problem to her professors: "I told them how I was feeling," she said. "Being honest with them made a bit of difference."

If you can control the influence of fatigue in your life, you may achieve the second goal: Keep fatigue from turning into exhaustion. Ignore the tasks that are unnecessary, and enlist help with those that are unavoidable.

If help is not forthcoming from one source, turn to another. Diane remembered disappointing exchanges with her mother-in-law: "His mother lived five minutes away, but she was like, 'It's hard. You gotta do it on your own. I have three kids, *I know how you feel.*'" This woman evidently feared that offering her daughter-in-law some help with an active one-year-old would rob her of the chance to build character. Do not, under any circumstances, subscribe to this belief yourself. Anything built on an exhausted foundation will only collapse at the first suggestion of stress. That's not the kind of home you want for your child. Instead, let yourself be raised, by the kind of cooperation that neighbors used to offer to raise each others' houses. After all, those structures built by the hands of the community have remained standing for a very long time.

5

Sleep Disturbances

PREGNANT WOMEN ARE, ON THE WHOLE, tired women. Hormonal changes produce fatigue and excessive sleepiness in the early weeks. Later, these effects are compounded by the effort of carrying excess weight and the loss of nighttime sleep, which tends to become increasingly restless, with more and more frequent awakenings. "Lately," wrote Dawn T. with a certain resignation in her seventh month, "a good night is when I get five or six hours and only have to get up every hour and a half." Linda Sue, also seven months pregnant, wrote:

> I am uncomfortable and therefore cannot sleep, or I wake up in discomfort (hip joint pain, backache, leg cramps). Also I have slight insomnia some nights, to the point that I dread bedtime because I don't relish tossing and turning for a couple of hours—but I'm too tired to do anything to occupy that time. I also find myself waking during the night with a start to wakefulness, and then I have great difficulty falling back to sleep. I've had very restless nights of late, and I'm prepared that it may just get worse in the next two months. I nap during the day to make up for the loss during the night. I'm *very* grateful to have that opportunity.

Any one or any combination of pregnancy's unique miseries may produce sleepless nights. Heartburn, leg cramps, night backache (or simply being unable to turn over in bed), urinary frequency, all possibly coupled with the needs of other children, can significantly disrupt sleep. "My son has just stopped waking up at night," sighed Linda B. as she embarked on her second pregnancy, "and now I have to get up to pee all the time." Unfortunately, Linda's experience is representative of the awful truth about sleep in pregnancy: Much of the time, you just can't win.

Sleep Disturbance Related to Posture

The main thing that can make sleep in pregnancy such a losing proposition is that no one has yet invented a good way to sleep standing up. A lot of pregnancy problems are simply worse when you're lying down—but "trying to sleep sitting up is about the *worst thing*," said Jae. "Sometimes I would lean over a whole bunch of pillows, but I never really could sleep that way. It was just miserable."

Heartburn. Jae's sleep was disrupted by heartburn, one of the worst offenders when it comes to sleep disturbance in pregnancy. To minimize the discomfort of heartburn, extra pillows are frequently recommended for raising the head, shoulders, and torso, but like Jae, many women find this an impossible position for sleeping. If you do use extra pillows, they must be adjusted so that the neck is not flexed forward. Try to get a ramp effect—a gradual upward slope—so that your back or neck is not kinked. Perhaps the best bet for a fairly comfortable night is a recliner, if you own one; if not, you may find yourself among the many who spend their late pregnancies trying to sleep sitting up on the living room couch, which certainly doesn't suggest a restful night. (For more information about heartburn see Chapter 6.)

Urinary frequency. At least one study has shown that the side-lying position interferes with the body's ability to concentrate urine, which means greater output because fluid reaches the bladder instead of being reabsorbed.[1] However, by the time you reach the second trimester, sleeping on your side is recommended by most OBs as the healthiest for you and the developing fetus, and it will probably be the most comfortable position as well. This puts you in another another can't-win situation. About the best you can do is to be as close to the bathroom as possible—even by using a chamber pot if you are upstairs and the only bathroom in the house is down. The less effort required to empty your bladder, the more likely you are to fall back to sleep easily.

Breathing disorders. If you sleep with someone who snores, you may already suspect that respiration is not always at its best during sleep. There are other circumstances that place stress on the respiratory system, and among these is pregnancy. Now imagine the respiratory system of a sleeping pregnant woman, and you begin to see the potential for problems.

Fortunately, in the great majority of pregnancies, sleep is not associated with serious breathing disorders or resulting problems for the fetus. However, the breathing difficulties sometimes produced by both the mechanical and the hormonal changes of pregnancy may result in an occasional uncomfortable night.

Probably the best way to prevent breathing problems in sleep is to stay off your back as much as possible in late pregnancy. By this stage, blood oxygenation decreases significantly when the mother is in a supine (back-lying) position. This position also increases the risk of obstructive sleep apnea (OSA), in which the sleeper's airway becomes closed for a number of seconds until the lack of oxygen awakens him, opening the airway and allowing breathing. This sequence of events may take place as many as fifty to one hundred times an hour all night long. The sleeper is unaware of the events and knows only that he never seems to feel rested. Our sleeper, by the way, is called *he* because the problem is most common in obese, middle-aged men.

Two factors theoretically place pregnant women at risk for OSA: the increased size of the abdomen, which might possibly cause problems normally associated with obesity, and the very common tendency toward nasal obstruction in pregnancy (see Chapter 8). However, studies have so far shown very few instances of OSA in pregnancy. Most recorded cases have occurred in obese women, so obesity likely is a significant risk factor, but the increased abdominal girth of normal pregnancy is probably not.

Though you will likely not suffer full-blown OSA, you may still feel that your breathing in sleep is uncomfortable or erratic. If so, simply placing some pillows behind you may prevent your rolling entirely onto your back and thus keep you more comfortable. Some women, especially those with nasal obstruction, also find their breathing is helped by elevating their heads, shoulders, and upper torsos with extra pillows. In other words, back to the recliner.

Night cramps. You have finally settled into a sound sleep when some psychopath plunges a knife deep into the calf of your leg. You sit bolt upright with a scream and clutch at the pain. The psychopath disappears, but the pain goes on as you massage a knot in your calf the size of a bantam's egg. This is a charley horse, a common enough occurrence in the general population and one to which you, as a pregnant person, are especially prone. In one study 60 percent of pregnant subjects complained of nocturnal leg cramps.[2] Many women interviewed for this book had the same complaint.

"I had nighttime feet and leg cramps," said Kim D. "It's like either my foot or my leg would all of a sudden try to fold itself in half. My big toe would shoot straight out and pull down and go *under* my foot. It was very strange to see (and quite painful)!"

"I had really bad leg cramps both times, near the end," said Diane. "Only at night in bed. It would be so bad that I would just about jump out of bed, and I would just lie there and scream and scream. I mean, I have never felt anything like that. They were terrible."

Jae said, "I would start to have them before I was conscious. So I would wake up screaming! And my husband would go, 'Aaaahhh! What's going on?' He was afraid the neighbors thought I was being beaten!" Like Jae, Linda Sue said her cramps were "severe enough to wake me with a start and bring me to tears. I am unable to walk until the cramp subsides."

Night cramps are associated with so many different conditions and circumstances–including (besides pregnancy) spinal disorders, cirrhosis, tetanus, defects of the central nervous system, even strychnine poisoning–that one explanation of their occurrence could not possibly account for all. There are certainly no agreements on why pregnant women suffer night cramps, which of course means no one can agree on the proper treatment, either.

Popular wisdom often blames leg cramps on a disturbed electrolyte balance, but sources disagree on which element is out of whack. Calcium deficiency is a popular theory, and one doctor claims that pregnant women's night cramps are often relieved by calcium supplementation.[3] However, many pregnant women are already supplementing calcium, with prenatal vitamin-mineral tablets (containing an average of 200 milligrams of calcium) and an almost feverish consumption of dairy products. It seems unlikely that all the pregnant women suffering night cramps could really be suffering calcium deficiency. Other sources claim that the cramps are caused by a lack of potassium and recommend a banana a day to keep cramps away. A third contingent points to sodium deficiency as the underlying factor, but as Doctor J. S. Black points out, even on a low-salt diet it is difficult for anyone to become truly salt deficient, as sodium occurs naturally in most foods.[4]

Dr. Black prefers to concentrate on the immediate precipitating factor, noting that leg cramps tend to occur when the leg is suddenly stretched. According to Dr. Black, when a woman sleeping on one side shifts to the other, she rolls onto her back, stretches her legs for a moment, and–zing! The attack of the knife-wielding psychopath.

Dr. Black recommends the simplest treatment imaginable: a pillow, placed under the covers at the foot of the bed (not behind the legs, which may hamper blood flow and thus create a risk of developing a clot). The pillow will prevent your fully stretching your legs and thus eliminate your leg cramps. Dr. Black claims a 100 percent cure rate over some ten years with this treatment, which certainly suggests that it's worth a try.

On the other hand, women who have had charley horses find that the right kind of stretching *relieves* the cramp. "If I would just stand up and go up and down on my tiptoes, they would go away," said Kim D. "Exercise and stretching help overall," noted Linda Sue. Ramsey said:

> I tell any woman that's just pregnant, "If you get the slightest cramp in your leg, *don't point your toes.*" This is something I learned the hard way. You know how you want to stretch in the morning, and you want to point your toes? Well, the thing you need to do instead is flex your foot back, bring your toes up toward your knee. As soon

as I would have the slightest feeling that I was going to get a cramp, I would do that, and it would alleviate the cramp.

Linda Sue agreed, saying that she experienced cramps not only at night but "while exercising, if I would forget and point my toes." Perhaps, then, the stretch in the night that brings on the cramp is a toe-pointing stretch. It is also possible that your foot may be forced into a toe point by tight covers at the bottom of the bed. Try loosening the covers or sleeping with your feet sticking out–but don't neglect your calcium supplement or your banana, either.

Restless legs. One of the strangest and most unpleasant nighttime complaints of pregnancy is the phenomenon of *restless legs*. The classic symptom is a crawling sensation in the legs (usually the lower legs, though the thighs may also be affected) that makes it impossible for the woman to keep her legs still. "Feels like bugs are crawling up and down my legs," wrote Linda Sue. "It still gives me the creeps to feel this sensation." Since the sensation is strongest when the legs are at rest, a woman may lose a lot of sleep as she spends most of the night moving her legs in an effort to quell the crawling feelings. Although the incidence of restless legs is slight among the general population (estimated 5 percent), the syndrome may effect veins in as many as one in every three pregnant women.

With so many potential subjects available, the syndrome would seem to lend itself to study, but it seems to be little researched and less understood. A recent paper offers a roundup of suggested associations and possible causes in the population at large: "heredity, depressive states, carcinoma, gastrectomy, infectious disease, varicose veins, cold amyloidosis, rheumatoid arthritis, and folic acid deficiency."[5] This offering hardly suggests that researchers are closing in on the cause, and except for speculation about folic acid levels (which should be normal in anyone taking prenatal vitamins), hardly even considers the circumstance of pregnancy. Treatment, too, has varied wildly: Doctors report relief of symptoms with a whole grab bag of drugs as well as vitamin C and the amino acid tryptophan. Though iron therapy has improved symptoms of restless legs in anemic patients, iron levels are already normal in most sufferers of restless legs syndrome. According to the paper already cited, "the majority of patients respond to simple explanation," though given the paucity of real information on the condition, it is hard to imagine how an explanation could be very satisfying. Remedies that may be of more use are massaging and pointing and flexing the feet. Doctors also suggest walking about, though you are probably spending enough time doing this while you want to be sleeping.[6]

If your life with restless legs has become truly impossible, you and your doctor may wish to consider some of the case reports on successful drug treatment. However, when confronted with a condition that apparently baffles the medical establishment, you may also wish to consider what an alternative practitioner such as a chiropractor might have to offer. A treatment that can't hurt and might help is often an attractive option for the sufferer of one of pregnancy's more infuriating (but harmless) conditions, and restless legs surely figures among these.

Night backache. Backache is a very common complaint in pregnancy (see Chapter 11), and for many women, the pain is worse at night. In one study, 67 percent of the subjects reported night backache, with 36 percent noting that the pain actually awakened them from sleep. The authors of this study note that, despite the apparent frequency of the complaint, night backache has received little attention from the medical community. Evidently, most health care providers are content with the two most common explanations for pregnancy-related backache: It is caused either by musculoskeletal stress resulting from weight gain or by the exaggerated curve of the pregnant woman's spine. Logically, however, neither of these theories pertains to a backache that occurs when a woman is lying down.[7]

The study cited proposes a mechanism for night backache that has nothing to do with gravity and everything to do with pregnancy, beginning with hormones. Those hormones produce changes in the veins of smooth muscles that greatly increase the capacity of uterine, ovarian, and pelvic blood vessels; in late pregnancy, ovarian veins may carry up to sixty times their normal capacity.

Given the tremendous volume of blood in the pelvic area, you might expect the rest of the circulatory system to be equally accommodating, but in fact it can be a tight squeeze. Ironically, even as pregnancy increases your blood volume, it develops a propensity to shut off the flow. The enlarged uterus can compress the *vena cava*, the large vein that carries blood from the lower part of the body back to the heart. When the vena cava is compressed, the blood must return to the heart through other, smaller vessels, many of them surrounding the lumbar vertebrae (the lower back). The effect is a lot like having a jackknifed trailer rig on your town's busiest freeway: The alternate routes get pretty congested. Furthermore, as you lie in bed, fluid that has accumulated in body tissues tends to move into the blood vessels, increasing the volume even more; so, to extend the freeway metaphor, you can think of your sleep time as rush hour for your circulatory system. If you spend that time flat on your back, the freeway—the vena cava—may be completely occluded for the entire length of your uterus. The resulting congestion in the blood vessels of the lower back causes swelling of these vessels and stagnation of the blood flow.

These are trying conditions for the dense tangle of nerve fibers that provides and receives impulses for these blood vessels. Both the excessive pressure and the stagnation (which prevents proper metabolism) may cause irritation of the nerves, resulting in lower back pain.

The fact that it takes some time for these conditions to build up explains why night backache may not develop until you have been asleep for some time. Of course, in some women it does not develop at all. The occurrence (or lack) of night backache probably depends on the extent of occlusion of the vena cava, the capacity of your "alternate routes" to handle the extra blood flow, and the amount of time you spend sleeping on your back (a position generally not recommended in late pregnancy).

By depriving nerves of a fresh blood supply, this same mechanism may also produce night cramps or restless legs (discussed earlier in this chapter). Everyone is familiar with the pins-and-needles feeling that comes when an unusual body position cuts off blood flow to the nerves of the foot or hand. Congested blood flow in the lower back may produce similar sensations within the legs. (The fact that these impulses are actually generated by the nerve fibers themselves explains why the feeling is perceived as deep within the legs.) The same congestion also produces electric potentials for involuntary muscular contraction, which may result in the stabbing pains of a charley horse.

If circulation rather than posture is truly responsible for nocturnal back pain in pregnancy, it might explain the failure of the popular belief that sagging mattresses produce aching backs. One study found no evidence of such a correlation; in fact, study subjects whose beds were slightly saggy actually slept better than those whose beds were not.[8]

In this study, women found the most relief from nighttime backache when their abdomens were supported (in the side-lying position) with a wedge-shaped pillow designed especially for the purpose. This pillow was curved to conform to the pregnant woman's shape, with a recessed portion into which the abdomen fits. Subjects in the study supported their abdomens with the special pillow for a week and with a standard pillow for a week. Subjects reported greater relief of backache with the special pillow; the relief seemed especially pronounced in women with more severe pain. However, it is worth noting that a number of the subjects rated both pillows helpful to some degree, so if you cannot procure a special pillow of some kind, your own pillow may still be of some help.

The authors of this paper also remark on the possibility that just taking part in the study may have increased some subjects' perceptions of improvement of their symptoms. They describe a "Hawthorne-like effect," referring to a depression-era study of lighting conditions at a Western Electric plant. In this study, workers' productivity improved when lighting was increased; however, it also improved when lighting was decreased. The morale boost came not from the lighting, but from being included in the study, which gave the workers the feeling that someone cared about their problems. In the case of the sleep study, the authors suggest that simply having their back pain and sleeping problems acknowledged might have resulted in some feeling of improvement in study subjects. Given the tendency of the medical community to ignore the "minor" discomforts of pregnancy, this suggestion is not far-fetched.

In fact, many of the journal articles frequently cited in studies of back pain in pregnancy seem to take the position that back pain is a norm to which all pregnant women should cheerfully adapt. One doctor noted that as far as many of his colleagues were concerned, pregnancy backache required "little more therapy than a certain amount of patience in listening to the patient describe the severity of her pain."[9] This description conjures up a picture of rolling eyes, stifled yawns, and surreptitious watch glances from the OB while the patient weeps with frustration over her disabling back pain. Small wonder that the women in the pillow study proved unusually faithful to the task of completing all the requirements of the study period. As the authors note, perhaps their enthusiastic participation demonstrated that the back pain of pregnancy "is not regarded as normal by those suffering from it" and that women "do not take it for granted" (as, the paragraph implies, doctors may do).

At any rate, here's hoping the pillow trick actually offers some balance and support to something besides your psyche. Anna recommends a body-length pillow:

> I couldn't have gotten through without those full-length body pillows. With those, I could lie on my side and put the pillow between my legs, and it would keep my legs separated. If my legs went together, it would squeeze my stomach too much, and I couldn't sleep. I started with one and I ended up with two of those pillows. I hemmed myself in. I had one on either side so I could just roll over.

Sources for these pillows include the Company Store (1-800-323-8000) and Spiegel (1-800-345-4500). Pillows aside, however, the benefits of finding a truly interested listener should not go unappreciated, whatever your pregnancy problem. Ideally that listener will be a health care provider of some sort, but if your doctor's idea of "a certain amount of patience" involves those surreptitious glances at the watch, be prepared to look elsewhere.

Changes in Sleep Patterns

Though firm conclusions as yet escape us (largely because of a scarcity of data in the field), there is at least reason to suspect that pregnancy alters the normal so-called architecture of sleep. That architecture involves predictable patterns of activity in the sleeping brain and body. Divided first into the two major categories of REM (rapid eye movement) and NREM (non-REM—that is, without eye movement) sleep, the patterns are further classified under NREM as Stages 1, 2, 3, and 4, according to brain activity measured by electroencephalograph (EEG).

The special characteristics of NREM sleep have earned it the name of *orthodox sleep* because it seems to offer the deep rest we all expect from a really good night's sleep. Though the muscles are not as relaxed as during REM sleep (when they become essentially paralyzed), the brain has descended into its deepest, slowest wave pattern, and all autonomic activity—the involuntary processes such as heart beat and respiration—is reduced, as are metabolic rates in both brain and body. In REM sleep, on the other hand, the brain seems almost hyperactive, and autonomic responses are similar to their wakeful states, despite the flaccid condition of the voluntary muscles.

Normal sleep begins with a period of *sleep latency*—the time between lights-out and actually falling asleep—after which the subject passes into NREM sleep, progressing through Stages 1 through 4, then moving into the first period of REM sleep. The sleeper will shift back and forth between NREM and REM sleep for the rest of the night, but Stage 3 and 4 sleep are usually limited to the early episodes of NREM.

The few existing EEG studies of sleep in pregnancy suggest that Stage 4 sleep is reduced, even absent, in the last trimester. This is certainly in keeping with the observation of greater wakefulness in late pregnancy, since Stage 4 is the "deepest" sleep state, while the other states move more toward wakefulness. (Consistent with this, the seemingly alert state of REM sleep appears to increase in the same period.)

Why might this be so? While urinary frequency or night backache might fracture sleep in a random way, the apparently consistent disruption of a particular sleep phase suggests a systemic influence rather than a localized physical discomfort. The fact that certain drugs can suppress specific phases of sleep is further evidence that changes in the brain's biochemical environment can lead to predictable changes in sleep patterns. Given the overload of hormones in pregnancy and the predilection of those hormones for rearranging all your accustomed neurochemistry, it makes sense to question their role in dismantling the architecture of sleep.

There is no question that the secretion of many hormones is related to the daily cycle of waking and sleeping hours. Studies have shown that most hormones exhibit circadian rhythms—that is, their levels in the blood rise or fall according to the time of day and whether the body is sleeping or awake. All this activity is regulated by the brain's so-called circadian pacemaker system. More and more, the folks who study these things (such as the American Sleep Disorders Association) are coming to believe that most sleep problems are a result of a circadian disturbance. The body clock, in other words, just isn't keeping correct time. In pregnant women, as in other sleep-disordered subjects, the evidence of such a disturbance includes measurable abnormalities in the secretion of certain hormones. Yet this evidence cannot settle the question of cause and effect. If hormonal secretion is altered by a disturbance of the pacemaker, what is the trigger for that disturbance? Most likely hormonal factors—and so we find ourselves chasing an answer around one of the many feedback loops that circle through the brain and body.

Still, we can set out on this circular journey from logical points, the first and most obvious being the reproductive hormones. Animal studies suggest that *neurotransmission,* chemical signaling in the brain, is heavily influenced by the sex steroids, including estrogens and progesterone. Among the daily functions that likely come under that influence is sleep. The effect of sex steroids on sleep is already familiar to sufferers of premenstrual syndrome. The fact that both oversleeping (hypersomnia) and insomnia are among the diagnostic criteria for PMS certainly suggests some hormonal basis for the regulation of the sleep cycles.

Though the precise mechanisms that initiate and maintain sleep are still largely a mystery, researchers have focused on the role of neurotransmitters. They have expended a good deal of effort in trying to determine whether a certain neurotransmitter or combination of neurotransmitters is responsible for the various sleep stages. Because there are different types of neurons, each responding to a specific neurotransmitter, researchers try to determine which type of *neuron* (nerve cell) is transmitting the signals appropriate to the given sleep stage. Studies demonstrate that action on the cholinergic neurons, for which acetylcholine is the neurotransmitter, are involved in producing and maintaining REM sleep. In contrast, actions on the adrenergic neurons, which signal through norepinephrine, seem to play at least some modulating role in inhibiting REM sleep. Unfortunately for our inquiry, NREM sleep has been less forthcoming with its secrets. However, since REM and NREM cannot occur simultaneously, perhaps it is reasonable to suspect that what inhibits REM may help to promote NREM. This suspicion casts an interesting light on the neurotransmitter norepinephrine.

Norepinephrine is a catecholamine, a neurotransmitter that stimulates the body and is secreted under stress. Perhaps because of its stimulatory properties, which include the ability to provoke uterine contractions, norepinephrine poses at least a theoretical risk to pregnancy. For this the body appears to compensate: As progesterone levels rise throughout pregnancy, norepinephrine levels appear to decline, or at least they have been shown to do so in animal studies. Researchers already suspect a link between progesterone and sleep disturbance; one study reported a decrease in Stage 4 in a subject who had received doses of progesterone,[10] and many papers note that sleep disruption in pregnancy is probably caused by high progesterone levels. Yet progesterone is also noted for its sedative effect. Perhaps, then, its disruptive action is specific to the mechanisms that produce Stage 4 sleep. Could it be that progesterone's apparent tendency to reduce levels of norephinephrine—a chemical that may help to promote NREM sleep—is in some way responsible for the lack of Stage 4 sleep in late pregnancy?

This hypothesis may have something in common with one theory of depression, which links that disorder to a deficiency (or perhaps inefficient use) of norepinephrine. Depression, in turn, is associated with sleep disorders—notably, a decrease or loss of Stage 4 sleep.

By now we are hurrying around our feedback loop again, for experimental suppression of Stage 4 sleep *produces* signs of depression in study subjects. Where is the cause, and where the effect? Does a depressed person lose Stage 4 sleep because he or she is in a biologically produced depression that alters sleep patterns as well as mood? Or does lack of sleep produce depression?

The few doctors who have studied sleep in pregnancy ask themselves the same questions. Depression is a common feature of pregnancy (see Chapter 3). When pregnant study subjects showed disturbances of Stage 4 sleep, was it a result of mild (and therefore undetected) depression? Or was Stage 4 sleep loss caused by hormonal changes that are also capable of producing depression? Whatever the answers, the tantalizing questions raised by the possibility of a three-way link between Stage 4 sleep loss, depression, and pregnancy ought to be causing researchers a few restless nights themselves.

Of course, pregnancy involves many other hormonal changes besides the increase of progesterone. With current research (almost none), it is impossible to say whether the changes have a direct action on the sleep cycle or reflect some other activity that is producing the disturbance.

Consider the steroid hormone cortisol. Cortisol is an arouser; among other stress-related duties, it helps to wake you up in the morning. Its secretion follows a very regular pattern, and more than half the cortisol your body produces in one twenty-four-hour cycle is released into the bloodstream in the early morning hours, as your regular rising time approaches.

High cortisol levels are associated with sleep disturbance, but the exact connection is unclear. It may be that the cortisol is not the cause of the disturbance, but a reflection of a stimulated state that breaks up the sleep cycle. A high level of cortisol in a nonpregnant person suggests intense activity in the *adrenal cortex*, part of the adrenal gland. It is quite possibly the adrenocortical activity, and not the cortisol itself, that produces sleep disturbance.[11]

The adrenal cortex secretes hormones vital to many of the functions that are greatly altered by pregnancy, including salt and water balance and the metabolism of fats, carbohydrates, and proteins. By the third trimester of pregnancy, concentrations of cortisol in the bloodstream are three times the nonpregnant level (so high that, outside of pregnancy, they would suggest a diseased state). While much of this increase is caused by a change in how cortisol is metabolized (the liver is slower to break it down), the adrenal cortex is also busy producing more of the steroid. The total effect suggests a system with enough activity to keep your whole neighborhood tossing in the sheets.

Actually, apart from any effect your stirrings may have on your bed partner, someone else may well be awake: the fetus. If the animal studies on pregnancy have any validity where humans are concerned, the fetal adrenal cortex is probably working overtime, too.

One of the primary animal subjects used in pregnancy studies is the sheep. In sheep, as term approaches, the fetal anterior pituitary releases increasing amounts of adrenocorticotropic hormone (ACTH), which stimulates the maturation of the fetal adrenal cortex. The adrenal cortex then releases a flood of cortisol, which is apparently key to the initiation of labor in sheep.

The differences between pregnancies in sheep and humans are wide indeed, and the findings from sheep studies are not always directly transferable to human beings. (Just for example, most of the cortisol in human fetal circulation comes from the mother, and cortisol does not appear to initiate labor.) Still, the evidence of intense adrenocortical activity in the late-gestation fetus holds up in primate studies. Could this activity affect the mother's sleep in some way? Just whose glands are keeping whom awake at night?

This brings us to the intriguing possibility that mother and fetus actually share sleep cycles. The sleep patterns of premature infants differ from those of full-term babies, which are different in turn from those of adults. One group of researchers monitored the sleep cycles of pregnant women and compared the results with the patterns commonly seen in premature infants. If you assume that sleep patterns of the premature infant resemble those of a fetus of the same gestational age, the suggestions of correlations between maternal and fetal sleep seem rather striking. For example, researchers recorded isolated movements of the mothers' eyes, different from the grouped movements seen in REM sleep, during NREM sleep Stages 2 and 3. Such movements are not normally seen in adults, but they are characteristic of infant sleep. Further, brain-wave readings showed that the mothers experienced spindles, a pattern of normal Stage 2 sleep, during REM sleep—again, an abnormal finding in an adult, but not unusual in a newborn. Spindle sleep in the appropriate stage (2) also increased in the mothers, but their Stage 2 sleep showed an unusual feature, now and then bursting out with periods of the slow waves normally seen in Stages 3 and 4. This, too, is a normal occurrence in newborn children. Finally, the sleep of the mothers resembled that of newborns in its lack of Stage 4, which does not develop in infants until some months after delivery, as well as in the increase of REM sleep at the end of pregnancy, characteristic of newborn sleep. After delivery, REM sleep decreases for both mother and child over a period of some eight weeks.[12]

The apparent similarities between maternal and fetal sleep suggest that sleep is regulated or affected by some factor transmissible in the blood–which leads us right back to hormones again. But who is pulling the hormonal trigger? Do the factors in question originate from the fetus, the placenta, or the mother? Evidence exists for each possibility. The intense activity of the fetal adrenal has already been discussed, as has the possible role of progesterone (placental origin) in sleep disturbance. Evidence for the role of maternal hormones comes from studies of nonpregnant women, which show alterations in sleep patterns following the changing levels of hormones throughout the menstrual cycle.

Most studies suggest that Stage 4 sleep returns quickly after delivery. This news may come as a surprise if you are not expecting to get *any* sleep, let alone four stages' worth, after your baby arrives. Consider, however, that because Stage 4 generally occurs in the first hours of sleep, you may reach that stage before your baby wakes up for the first night feeding. In fact, while total sleep time will almost certainly decrease after delivery, a greater amount of that time will be spent in Stage 4, suggesting that the mother of the newborn at least gets the most possible rest from the least time in bed.

On the other hand, some women experience insomnia after delivery, marked by the continued absence of Stage 4 sleep. For at least a hundred years, such insomnia has been associated with the disorder known as *postpartum psychosis*, in which the mother suffers serious psychiatric illness some two weeks after an apparently uneventful delivery. So commonly is this illness preceded by insomnia that doctors are advised to take very seriously all complaints of sleeplessness in the postpartum period. Though many a mother may feel that waking up every two hours to nurse a new baby is driving her crazy, these normal interruptions of sleep are not likely the cause of postpartum psychosis. Insomnia arises from within, not from outside interruptions. It is the inability to sleep even when given the chance. It seems more likely that sleep disturbance postpartum, particularly the continued absence of Stage 4 sleep, might represent a failure of hormones to make the normal adjustments after delivery. A mother may thus be left in a compromised state, at risk for depression or other psychiatric illness.

In view of the evidence–such as it is–there seems good reason to believe that sleep disturbance in pregnancy, apart from bathroom trips and backache, has a hormonal basis. Whether that indicates some sort of biological reasoning is much less clear. It's tempting to jump at the explanation that the loss of deep sleep somehow prepares mothers for the coming months of nighttime infant care. Maybe they become accustomed to lack of sleep, or (as subjects in one study reported) they are more easily awakened by sounds that never interrupted their sleep before pregnancy, or perhaps the apparent synchronicity of their sleep cycles with their infants *in utero* will continue after birth. These are all attractive theories, but hard to reconcile with existing studies, most of which suggest that the mother's sleep cycles return to normal rather quickly following delivery.

Those studies, however, are very few, and many of them were carried out with the tiniest samples imaginable (often only four or five subjects), making their observations interesting but hardly statistically sound. The fact is that the data are currently too scarce to determine *if* pregnancy produces predictable sleep disturbances, let alone *why*. Perhaps with more extensive studies, researchers could make more sense out of sleep patterns in pregnancy.

Then again, there is much about the experience of pregnancy that seems to bugger explanation, and it may be too romantic a view of nature to believe that every symptom has been engineered to benefit the mother and child. If this were true, wouldn't they be universally suffered? Instead, they are distributed through the population in a random way, suggesting that they are more likely caused by individual reactions to hormones, as varied and unpredictable as responses to drugs or even foods. Some of the reactions may result in problems that are in no way beneficial to either mother or child (postpartum psychosis being an obvious example).

There is even evidence suggesting that other hormones attempt to compensate for disturbed sleep. Melatonin, a hormone vitally connected to the body's adjustments to night and day, is present in high levels in women who sleep poorly in late pregnancy. Researchers have speculated that since melatonin has demonstrated hypnotic properties, its release is probably not causing the sleep disturbances but is more likely the body's attempt to counteract them.[13]

Perhaps sleep disturbances and other pregnancy symptoms are the remnants of evolutionary traits from which we once benefited and with which we are now simply stuck, like wisdom teeth. (Of course, you can have wisdom teeth removed.)

Whatever the case, women really would benefit from knowing whether sleep disturbance in pregnancy can or even should be treated. Anyone who doubts the importance of these questions should reread the history of Thalidomide, a drug marketed as a sedative in Europe between 1953 and 1961. The widespread use of this drug by pregnant women—which became tragically apparent when many infants were born with severe limb deformities—demonstrates that large numbers of women were disturbed enough by their sleep problems to discuss them with their doctors and to accept a prescription for a sleeping aid. While the attitude toward using such drugs in pregnancy has changed since the Thalidomide tragedy, there is no reason to think that women are sleeping any better. Likely they are simply accepting the disturbances with more stoicism.

Some relief, fortunately, may be possible without drugs. "What helped me the most," wrote Louise, "was my husband taking me through a progressive relaxation exercise, from head to toe." Relaxation exercises are one of the great remedies for many pregnancy complaints. They may involve guided imagery, in which a live or taped coach leads you through a series of relaxing images. They may involve deliberate tensing and then release of the muscles, usually in a toe-to-head progression. Good resources for learning such exercises include hypnotherapists, clinical psychologists, or purchased books or tapes.

Other effective nondrug remedies may exist, but lack of research so far prevents their use. If sleep disturbance in pregnancy could be conclusively attributed to disruptions of the circadian rhythm, women might benefit from therapies already proven effective in similar circumstances, such as bright light therapy (see Chapter 3) or vitamin B12 supplementation. The ideal, of course, would be first to establish whether alterations of sleep cycles in pregnancy are a beneficial mechanism—in which case most mothers would suffer them gladly—or simply a coincidental effect.

However, if the current state of research indicates current interest and support, we'll have to hope for answers in our dreams.

6

Heartburn

"THEY NEED A NEW DESCRIPTION FOR THIS," said Dawn T. "'Heartburn' doesn't cut it." At about five months, Dawn began experiencing attacks of intense pain that started behind the breastbone, radiated up into her shoulders, and then moved down into her abdomen. "It would begin and end very suddenly," she wrote, "and last anywhere from three to fifty minutes. It was incapacitating. I would have to go into the bathroom at work and wait for it to go away. The pain made me break out in a sweat."

Dawn was skeptical of her obstetrician's diagnosis of heartburn—"I told him it was *not* gastric. It had to be something else, it was so painful"—but she tried the antacid Mylanta after every meal as he recommended. "It worked," she said, and in her sixth month of pregnancy noted that she was still taking it: "I go through a bottle every two weeks now."

This is heartburn—not as many popular and professional works describe it ("a mild to moderate pain") but as some pregnant women really experience it. "A really hot, sore spot," said Kim D.,

> . . . about the size of my fist, and it sits right at the bottom of my breastbone. . . . It was so bad and so clearly defined, it was as if I could just pull it out. It honestly was like a baseball . . . and it was on *fire!* I feel as if I've never had heartburn before, if that was what it was. The pain didn't radiate up, but down—along the sides of my big belly—but there was still a very definite starting point. I have never had a pain like that in my life. I'm getting ghost pain right now, just thinking about how bad it was.

Researchers have always claimed, with great conviction, to understand the cause of pregnancy heartburn. The fact that what they "know" to be true has changed every ten years or so has not lessened their confidence. Yet even the most up-to-date research seems insufficient to explain the type of pain Kim and Dawn describe, with its intensity, its definition, and (in Dawn's case) its abrupt beginning and ending. Assuming that it was heartburn—as Dawn's relief from antacids at least seems to suggest—how do their cases fit in with current perceptions regarding this common pregnancy complaint?

Until about 1970, pregnancy heartburn was primarily viewed as a problem of body mechanics: The enlarging uterus, by compressing the stomach, increases gastric pressure. According to this logical theory, the increased pressure forces the stomach contents (made acid by their stay in the stomach) backward through the lower esophageal sphincter (LES), up into the esophagus where the pressure is lower. This reflux, or backward motion of partially digested food, is assumed to cause the burning discomfort of heartburn.

This is not a bad theory as far as it goes, and it still enjoys wide circulation. However, research soon began to suggest a more complicated picture. One study showed that in men suffering ascites, a condition that produces gastric pressure similar to that of pregnancy, the LES actually compensated for the additional gastric pressure with increased pressure of its own.[1] Apparently in nonpregnant people the LES is normally capable of preventing reflux by adjusting its own pressure as stomach pressure increases.

But further research turned up evidence that the function of the LES is probably compromised by the hormones of pregnancy. Studies found that many pregnant women—even some without symptoms of heartburn—demonstrated lower LES pressure than nonpregnant women and that the pressure continued to fall as pregnancy progressed. Researchers suspected progesterone might cause this change in pressure, since progesterone in general decreases muscle tone, but apparently a combination of estrogens and progesterone is required. Once pregnancy had set this effect into motion, nothing could increase LES pressure—not drugs, not hormones, not food—until delivery. So by the 1980s, this reduced LES pressure took over as the primary acknowledged cause of reflux in pregnancy, in combination with the mechanical changes noted earlier. Studies since then have continued to support the idea that pregnancy hormones play a role, as in one paper reporting that increasing severity of pregnancy heartburn corresponded more to increasing progesterone levels than to the mechanical effect of the growing uterus.[2]

However, in the most recent papers on pregnancy heartburn, low LES pressure seems to be losing its status as the principle mechanism allowing reflux. Researchers are at last beginning to regard reflux in pregnancy as a complex condition involving many factors—a view always worthy of applause, since it suggests increasing respect for the pregnant body as a complicated system instead of a bag of separately misbehaving parts. At any rate, recent research puts LES pressure in a different perspective. A study of gastrointestinal reflux in the general population[3] demonstrated that reflux does not occur continually, as a consistently low LES pressure would suggest, but during brief episodes when the LES relaxes altogether. These relaxations are apparently controlled by the *vagus nerve*, which carries sensory information from the esophagus. (Vagal nerve pathways run through neck, chest, and abdomen and extend to most of the major organs, which probably explains why esophageal pain can radiate up and down the body.) Thus the relaxations may be provoked by stimuli inside the esophagus that send messages to the vagus nerve. The idea that LES actions are neurally controlled seems to cast some doubt on the importance of decreased muscle tone.

Further, heartburn does not necessarily follow every episode of reflux. The occurrence and severity of heartburn likely depend on how long the refluxed contents stay in the esophagus, irritating the tissue and probably causing a supersensitivity of pain receptors there. The esophagus has its own mechanism for clearing these irritating substances, but this wave-motion mechanism, like the motion of the intestines, appears to be slowed or impaired by hormones in pregnancy. So we're back to progesterone and the estrogens, but focused on a different site, the esophagus itself.

In fact, one textbook on gastrointestinal disease distinguishes between heartburn and esophageal pain. The latter is also a burning pain with the same location and the same tendency to radiate, but "the pain episodes may last for minutes to hours. . . . The pain can be severe, causing the patient to become ashen and perspire. Symptoms often abate spontaneously."[4] This sounds more like what Dawn T. sweated out in the restroom at work—and this pain is even less understood than heartburn. According to the textbook, it may be provoked by distention of the esophagus, which could produce pain by activating "stretch receptors." It may also be true that disordered motility—problems with the motion of the esophagus—is caused by the pain rather than bringing on the pain as has been assumed with heartburn. It could also be that symptoms occur because the pain threshold has been altered in some way.(Study subjects with no symptoms of esophageal pain can tolerate more stretching of the esophagus.) Antidepressant medications that raise the pain threshold have reduced esophageal pain even when no obvious change occurred in the action of the esophagus. To date there has been no research on whether pregnant women might actually be suffering this type of chest pain rather than garden-variety heartburn.

All this squabbling and trumping in thirty years' worth of medical literature may seem like academic trivia if you're sleeping upright on the sofa with a bottle of Mylanta in your hand, but there really is a point to it all. Real understanding of pregnancy ailments is vital to treatment decisions. Without understanding, it is impossible even to guess how any symptom relates to the pregnancy. Is it a reflection of some process vital to the maintenance of the pregnancy—in which case "treatment" would be the last thing you'd want—or a by-product that you, the innocent bystander in a hormonal riot, can treat symptomatically? And what treatments are appropriate?

The most recent papers on pregnancy heartburn, with their focus on acid buildup and tissue damage over time, suggest that symptoms are cumulative. If that is the case, symptoms might be avoided or at least lessened by early preventive measures. Some studies indicate that reflux often begins early in pregnancy, but women do not always notice the symptoms until later (which supports the buildup theory). Though data conflict, there are also some suggestions that certain factors put some women at risk for heartburn. Among these are numerous pregnancies and heartburn symptoms experienced before pregnancy. (Despite what you may have heard, weight gain and prepregnancy weight do not appear to correlate with heartburn prevalence.) So if you have a history of heartburn, or of childbearing, or of heartburn while childbearing, you might especially want to take action before symptoms appear or become severe.

Mechanical therapies. Even in early pregnancy, it may help to avoid positions that set the mechanical causes of heartburn in motion. For instance, the most common prescription for heartburn is elevation of the head and shoulders during sleep. If you begin this simple therapy early in pregnancy, it may decrease the severity of heartburn in the later months. You can also avoid positions that invert your insides, such as bending at the waist (while you still *can* bend at the waist).

Adjusting eating habits. Keeping your meals small and frequent may also help from the beginning—though this standard prescription is probably meaningless for most pregnant women, who tend either to eat all the time or to be unable to eat anytime, regardless of the doctor's advice.

Lisa, who suffered progressively worsening heartburn from about five weeks through term, said that it got so bad she *couldn't* eat:

> I lost eight to ten pounds in the last month of my pregnancy. The thought of trying to eat was so unpleasant. You could smell [the sour stomach] on my breath. It felt like there was no room at all in my tummy.

Many times, the only thing Lisa could put in her stomach was "cool water. Maybe I just felt like it helped, maybe it was more a psychological aid, but it felt like it cooled it."

Still, many women find that eating helps the heartburn, at least temporarily. This makes sense in the context of LES pressure, which is highest after a meal and when the stomach is most active. Eating the right thing at the right time may provide some relief, as Kim D. wrote:

> The heartburn started fairly early, but it was very mild [at first]. I believed it to be an upset stomach at first. I would drink ice water and eat crackers and it seemed to help. It did show up most when I was hungry, but it wouldn't go away completely for about twenty-four hours. Then, I had to be careful not to get really hungry again, for fear it would come back. Believe it or not, very cold lemonade helped. It sounds disgusting, but it helped more than anything else!

Noting that antacids didn't offer much relief when the pain was really severe, Kim added, "Usually sleep would help, or eating a small, very mild food, like a plain flour tortilla with lemonade."

Eating also produces saliva, and saliva helps to neutralize and clear acid from the esophagus. In fact, if every now and then your mouth suddenly fills with a clear, slightly salty fluid (called *water brash*), this is quite possibly a sign that your body is trying to combat acid in the esophagus. To bring on salivation when you don't feel like eating, you may find it helpful to chew gum or suck hard candies.

When you do eat, be careful. Certain foods have been associated with heartburn, probably either because they actually lower LES pressure or because they irritate the esophagus directly (a property that is apparently independent of acidity, so the traditional prescription of eating a bland diet is not precisely appropriate). Foods that reduce esophageal sphincter pressure include fats, chocolate, and peppermint. Direct irritants include citrus, tomatoes, spicy foods, and coffee. Unfortunately, reactions to food also seem to be fairly individual, so you may never know what's going to hit you until you are already incapacitated, as Dana remembered:

> Mine was salmon croquettes. I called my cousin and asked for a recipe. She read it to me over the phone, and I cooked it. That night I could not lie down, the pain was so bad, and I thought, "I am going to *die* of indigestion." It was like, that day I quit throwing up and started having indigestion, and it was as miserable as the nausea.

Even the order in which you eat things may affect your symptoms, according to Linda Sue, who also had heartburn throughout her pregnancy. She offered one of her midwife's suggestions that proved somewhat effective: "Drink liquids thirty minutes after meals instead of with." The theory is that liquids consumed with the meal cause the stomach's more solid contents to float upward, increasing backward pressure on the esophagus.

Medication. If you do need medication, the good news is that most heartburn medications are *nonsystemic*—that is, they work directly on the affected site (stomach or esophagus) instead of spreading through the bloodstream—and so are assumed safe in pregnancy. However, they may not prove equally effective for you, so you may have to shop around. Some may even be unbearable, as Lisa remembered: "My doctor told me to take Gaviscon, but it was so foamy and thick I couldn't swallow it without gagging. It was almost as bad as the heartburn." Lisa, like many pregnant women, became something of a Tums addict. (When Dana described Tums as a "daily thing," Jae laughed and amended, "Hourly thing!")

Over-the-counter antacids such as Mylanta are widely prescribed for heartburn in pregnancy, and studies do not show any connection between antacids and birth defects, even with daily doses. Doctors generally recommend using them after meals and before bedtime. There is one cautionary note: Antacids may interfere with the absorption of iron.

Heartburn remedies that are based on sodium bicarbonate (such as Alka-Seltzer) should *not* be taken in pregnancy because they may cause imbalance of fluids or disturb the blood pH in either mother or fetus.

A recent review[5] offers several suggestions for physicians regarding prescription drugs to use or to avoid for pregnancy heartburn. A summary of these suggestions, which you may wish to discuss with your doctor in choosing heartburn medication, follows:

Name/Brand Name/Comments

Sucralfate/Carafate/Provided significant relief to study subjects. Essentially none of this drug is absorbed by the body, making it the preferred prescription drug for pregnancy heartburn.

Metoclopramide/Not studied for efficacy in treating pregnancy-related heartburn.

Cimetidine/Tagamet/Crosses placenta. Not well studied in humans. Anecdotal reports of problems have not been conclusively linked to drug, but women may wish to avoid in pregnancy.

Ranitidine/Zantac/Crosses placenta. Very few case reports of pregnancy outcomes. Reports that do exist show no adverse outcomes but do not state whether drug was effective for mothers' symptoms.

The authors of this report counsel against the use of three other drugs: famotidine (Pepcid), nizatidine (Axid), and omeprazole (Prilosec). Of the former two there are no reports on use in pregnancy, and the latter has been shown to produce birth defects in animals.

Finally, turning from medical writing to the Old Wives' Tales Department: If you are experiencing the kind of heartburn Kim D. and Dawn T. describe, folklore holds that your baby will be born with a lot of hair. This held true for all subjects interviewed for this book, like Kim, who had heartburn only in her second pregnancy and noted that while her first baby was bald until eighteen months, her second was born with hair that "covered the tops of her ears and curled along the nape of her neck." You might as well get those itty-bitty combs and brushes ready. You could arrange them on the bathroom shelf, right between the Mylanta bottle and the six-pack of Tums. Happy brushing!

7

Bell's Palsy

A GOOD EXAMPLE OF PREGNANCY'S ABILITY to produce the most alarming symptoms is Bell's palsy, a facial nerve disorder of sudden onset that occurs in perhaps one in 2,600 pregnancies. Typically, a woman might wake up one morning with virtually complete paralysis of one side of her face. She will have difficulty even closing her eye on that side, and a number of her senses may be affected—taste may be lost, and hearing on the affected side may be either decreased or painfully sensitive to loud noises. Her ears may ring. She may drool or even have slurred speech.

Most women are aware that pregnancy is associated with blood pressure changes and that in some women those changes carry a risk of stroke. Naturally, then, the sudden onset of symptoms that most people associate with stroke can be alarming, even terrifying, to the pregnant woman. However, in most cases, the diagnosis will be Bell's palsy. While this disorder occurs in the general population, its incidence is approximately three times higher among pregnant women, particularly in the last trimester.

Bell's palsy is a lower motor neuron paralysis of the facial nerve (the seventh cranial nerve, for anyone who might be counting); the onset is sudden and the cause is unknown. The disorder was named for Sir Charles Bell, a surgeon practicing in the early nineteenth century. In 1830, Bell noted an apparent increase in this condition in pregnant women, an observation that has been supported by many physicians since then.

Bell's palsy may also occur just after birth, as in Sally's case. Sally began experiencing ringing and roaring of the ears in about her seventh month. Such ear complaints are common in pregnancy (see Chapter

8), but they have also been reported early in the course of Bell's palsy. Sally wrote:

> After my baby was born, the [ear] symptoms got worse. I stayed in the hospital for a full week, not for the baby but for me. I lost my balance a few times and just felt strange and awful, in spite of my euphoric state. After a week, I begged to go home. It was my birthday, and we had family over to celebrate both birthdays. At dinner, I felt my mouth was drooping and asked my husband about it. He couldn't see anything, but sent me to bed. I awoke to feed the baby and discovered I could not move the entire right side of my face. I literally screamed, "I've had a stroke, and no one's been listening to me!" But the words didn't even sound right, because only the left side of my mouth would move. My right eye wouldn't shut, either. I was a sight!

Because pregnancy-related cases of Bell's tend to cluster in the last trimester, most researchers have focused on the physical circumstances of that period in their attempts to find a cause for the disorder. A popular theory focuses on fluid retention, which is at its peak during those last months. According to this theory, fluid retention and tissue swelling around the facial nerve cause nerve compression. A similar mechanism is often proposed for other pregnancy-related ailments such as carpal tunnel syndrome (see Chapter 12).

Other hypotheses connect Bell's, via various mechanisms, to hypertension in pregnancy. This hypertension might contribute to increased fluid retention, which takes us right back to the explanation above; or it could affect the facial nerve by changing its blood supply, if a blood vessel near the nerve were to develop even a very small clot. However, studies attempting to associate Bell's with hypertension have produced conflicting results, some supporting an association, and others finding none. It is certain, at any rate, that the condition is not limited to women with hypertensive pregnancies.

Some hypotheses focus on how the altered immune system of a pregnant woman might allow a reactivation of a dormant virus, which could then affect the facial nerve. The herpes group of viruses are notorious for their ability to lie dormant in the body for years. In late pregnancy, the immune system is increasingly suppressed, and a virus such as *herpes simplex* may be reactivated. Another virus in this group, *herpes zoster*, is known to affect the facial nerve in a condition called Ramsay-Hunt syndrome. It seems possible that a herpes virus could be at work in Bell's palsy, and indeed, Bell's patients in several studies have shown a level of antibodies to the herpes group that is significantly higher than in the general population. In one study 100 percent of the Bell's palsy patients showed evidence of previous infection with herpes simplex.[1]

Whatever the cause, the prognosis for a patient with Bell's palsy is usually very good. Most people recover quickly and spontaneously, many of them within two weeks of the onset of symptoms.

This was not the case for Sally, who described her struggle with Bell's and her course of treatment as "a ride on an endless roller coaster." She went on:

> I had a wonderful doctor who treated me with Prednisone and diuretics and shared my tears on my biweekly hookups to the electrode machine to ensure the facial nerve was alive. He told me I had 100 percent paralysis and we had to be careful the nerve wasn't permanently damaged.
>
> At any rate, I slowly progressed, though it took a year to get to the point that I am right now. I still have some residual problems, but most people can't see them, and I know how lucky I am. Dorothy was the perfect infant. Somehow she knew I was having problems and she was easy on me. Of course, after I was totally well, and she was eighteen months, she paid me back!

The use of diuretics Sally described is based on the fluid retention–nerve compression theory. Some doctors caution that the use of diuretics in treating Bell's palsy has not been well studied.[2] Because she was treated after pregnancy, Sally could also receive the oral steroids often prescribed to nonpregnant Bell's patients. These, too, are assumed to reduce swelling around the nerve. However, because such therapy carries at least a theoretical risk of complications or birth defects, it might not be the treatment of choice for a pregnant patient. Instead, many doctors feel that in most cases, the likelihood of spontaneous recovery weighed against the unproved effectiveness and theoretical risks of both diuretics and steroids argues for a conservative, wait-and-see approach to the the pregnant Bell's patient. During that period of waiting and seeing, a doctor might suggest eye drops if eye muscle weakness leads to dryness. Some doctors also recommend massage of the facial muscles, to stimulate nerve endings as well as to relax the nonaffected muscles, which may tense in an attempt to compensate for the partial paralysis.

For Sally, the course of Bell's was unusually long-lasting and severe. Still, "nearly nine years later," she wrote, "I can honestly say I'd go through it all again to have my daughter."

8

Ear, Nose, Throat, and Mouth Problems

By their third or fourth month, many women have come to think of pregnancy as an uncontrollable force whose presence may manifest itself anywhere in their bodies at any time. Still, when a woman notices she has been through twelve boxes of Kleenex and still can't breathe through her nose, she is more likely to blame colds or allergies than to think of that alien life force; when the members of her church choir suggest that she give up her soprano chair for a space in the tenors, she will probably just assume she's been pushing herself too hard and talking too much in an attempt to get all her work done before that alien becomes a real baby. Nevertheless, problems with nose and throat are quite common in pregnancy—perhaps nearly universal; it is hard to estimate the occurrence of symptoms that few women are likely to connect with the pregnancy. (Some one-third of pregnant women may report the symptoms to their doctors.) Most of these problems are assumed to be the result of pregnancy-related changes in the tissue of the nasal passages and connecting structures. Because those structures include the upper part of the pharynx into which the eustachian tubes open, the ears are also affected.

As you are no doubt aware by now, pregnancy involves tremendous fluid retention. That fluid is retained just about everywhere, including the mucous membranes of the nose and throat. The resulting swelling of these membranes is perhaps the primary change that leads to other problems. Also, those powerful hormones that have laid waste to the rest of your life are making their mark on your breathing as well. In animal studies, estrogens have been found to increase both the thickness of the mucous membranes and the number of blood vessels they contain. They also produce swelling of the tissue lining the smallest blood vessels of the nose, causing them to thicken as well.

The size of blood vessels in the nose is also controlled by nerves (in what is called a *vasomotor reaction*). These nerve responses are brought about by the effects of *acetylcholine*, the chemical transmitter that sends nerve impulses to muscle fibers. Normally, when this chemical is released from nerve endings, it is broken down almost immediately. In the presence of estrogens, however, this deactivation is slowed. With acetylcholine more available to act on the nerves, the vasomotor response is exaggerated.

Immune reactions may also be involved. Some researchers believe that women may respond to placental or fetal proteins with nasal allergic symptoms. One group concentrated on a substance known as *vasoactive intestinal polypeptide* (VIP). Nerves that produce swelling as an immune reaction to this substance exist in the nasal membranes of some animals (and in the genitals of the human male, where they are assumed to play a role in erection). Since progesterone and oxytocin are known to release VIP in the gastrointestinal tract of humans, VIP as a cause of nasal congestion in pregnancy is at least theoretically possible, though the measurements used in the first test of this hypothesis did not produce supportive findings.[1]

The condition of the nasal membranes in pregnancy must be very inviting to opportunistic infections–an assumption supported by the fact that many pregnant women experience excruciating sinus infections, or colds that never seem to end. Ramsey, who suffered sinusitis in two pregnancies, noted that such infections have an impact on much more than the nasal passages:

> The infections just accentuated everything about pregnancy. I was already feeling run-down, drained, from morning sickness. So with the sinus infections, my whole health was really down. And then I had to worry about taking medications, which you hate to do because you assume there is some risk with anything you take.

At least in the second pregnancy, Ramsey had one aid on hand: "A diaper in every room," she said, for continuous nose blowing. Ramsey did take antibiotics for the infections, even resorting to a second prescription in the second pregnancy after the first prescription proved ineffective. She evaluated all prescriptions carefully with her physician before agreeing to take them, as should any pregnant woman whose doctor suggests an antibiotic. Remember that while antibiotics cannot cure a cold (which is a virus and thus not susceptible to antibiotics), given the right conditions–such as mucous membranes nicely primed by pregnancy–a virus can open the door to a bacterial infection. If your cold from hell has lasted for most of your trimester, check with your doctor. While you may be understandably hesitant to medicate yourself at the first sign of a sniffle, preferring to bear the symptoms and avoid the risk, a sinus infection that seriously compromises your health and well-being does not do your baby any good, either.

Though it may be hard to tell where viruses or bacteria leave off and allergies begin, some women suffer nasal allergies for the first time during pregnancy. Women previously troubled by allergies may find them exacerbated. Then again, some women with a history of nasal allergic symptoms experience *relief* of those symptoms while pregnant. Like many other complaints, the varied course of allergy in pregnancy exemplifies the highly individual nature of each body's reaction to pregnancy.

Those lucky enough to experience relief are likely benefiting from the fact that pregnancy, especially in the last trimester, is an immunosuppressed state. As pregnancy progresses, the steroid hormone cortisol is produced in steadily rising amounts. (At term, the level of cortisol in the mother's blood is three times the nonpregnant levels.) Cortisol suppresses the immune system by lowering the level of lymphocytes circulating in the blood. Because cortisol has anti-inflammatory properties, it also reduces the inflammatory response. This reduction accounts for the improvement of allergy symptoms in some women. However, the lowered immune response may leave a woman at risk for viral infections or for the reactivation of infections (such as viruses in the herpes group) that have lain dormant in the body, so what a mother-to-be gains in allergy relief she may lose in the battle against a whole host of bugs.

If you go to your doctor with a nose that feels stuffy, drips a thin, watery discharge, is red from constant blowing and wiping and swollen within and without; if you also complain of feelings of facial fullness or tenderness; and if you tell this doctor that you have experienced these symptoms since your third month and are still suffering in your seventh, you may be diagnosed with neither sinusitis nor allergy but simply *rhinitis of pregnancy*. The swollen nasal membranes can easily produce these symptoms even in women with no infection or environmental irritants. Many of these women, assuming that they are suffering a one- or two-day cold, medicate themselves with over-the-counter preparations—an unfortunate choice that only exacerbates their symptoms. The hormonally influenced dilation and swelling of the nasal membranes strongly resists topical medications such as nose drops or sprays. A woman using these may experience brief relief, but a rebound effect will soon make the stuffiness worse. In many cases, the woman will then try more nose drops and sprays, which make the problem worse than ever. At the point when she finally gives up and goes to the doctor, this woman will likely have *rhinitis medicamentosa*—that is, she has medicated herself into severe inflammation.

To avoid this ailment, it is a good idea to stay away from nasal sprays and drops in pregnancy. Furthermore, anything taken in through the nasal membranes is rapidly absorbed throughout the body, so you need to consider the possibility of more than the nose being subject to the effects of the medication. With oral decongestants, too, there is a risk that their effect (constriction of the swollen vessels, which offers a feeling of relief) can be produced systemwide. Theoretically, this systemic effect could cause insufficient blood supply to the placenta, though the literature notes that this theory has not been supported by data. Whatever the case, it is certainly best to talk to your doctor before taking any over-the-counter medication for nasal symptoms in pregnancy.

A pregnant woman with miserable symptoms knows how far the reality of pregnancy can differ from the gauzy, glowing image presented in advertising–and a prime example is the woman whose pregnancy brings a sudden onslaught of nosebleeds. There is nothing like having your nose spout blood over the bows and ruffles on your maternity dress to bring reality home. Nosebleeds in pregnancy are not uncommon. Because most of them likely result from changes in the nasal mucosa and the congested state of the blood vessels in the nose, most bouts with nosebleeds can be expected to resolve when the nasal tissue returns to normal, if not before; that is, the condition generally limits itself.

Nosebleeds can also be a sign of a rare type of nasal obstruction that arises during pregnancy called *nasal granuloma gravidarum*. A granuloma is a benign growth, and gravidarum simply means a condition occurring in the gravid, or pregnant, woman. Symptoms of a nasal granuloma include nosebleeds and nasal obstruction, both of which will become worse as the growth increases in size. If the growth is large enough, you may feel the mass itself inside your nostril.

Some doctors believe that these growths are caused when the nasal tissue, congested and full of tiny new blood vessels from the changes occurring in pregnancy, suffers some other trauma. Irritations produced by cold weather may be sufficient, or a growth might result from some minor injury resulting from nose blowing or picking.

How a nasal growth of this nature is treated depends on the symptoms and the stage of pregnancy. Recent literature suggests that if a patient is close to term, has only minor bleeding and obstruction of the nose, and is carefully observed by her doctor for any changes, she can wait until after delivery to have the growth removed. Profuse bleeding will likely require more immediate action, particularly if the woman is not very close to her due date.[2]

In either case, the common practice is to remove these growths under local anesthesia. Brief hospitalization may be included, to insure that the blood flow has stopped. Whether the growth will recur is apparently not predictable. Some cases have involved more than one repeat performance while others have had no recurrence.

Changes in the nose and throat area in pregnancy can also lead to problems with the ears, largely through the eustachian tubes, which run from the middle ear to open into the back of the throat and provide for the flow of air in and out of the middle ear. Eustachian tube dysfunction in pregnancy appears to be another of those highly individual reactions: Some women experience obstruction, while in others the tubes will be abnormally open (patulous).

Sally had classic symptoms of eustachian tube dysfunction starting about her seventh month:

> I began suddenly to have tinnitus (ringing in the ears) and my ears seemed to be forever stopped up (like the feeling you get in airplanes). Once when I was on a business phone call, the tinnitus was so bad I had to hang up. One night, I awoke frightened that someone was stomping through the house, only to realize it was the sound of my heartbeat in my ears.

Sally's symptoms may have been connected with her later bout with Bell's palsy (see Chapter 7). Some doctors theorize that both problems are caused by the edema of pregnancy. Certainly the occurrence of eustachian tube problems is correlated with nasal congestion.

Symptoms of eustachian tube obstruction resemble the feeling you get, as Sally described, on airplanes, or as Linda Sue described it, "like I'm changing altitudes when I'm doing *nothing*." Like most women, Linda Sue complained of fullness and popping (other frequent complaints are muffling of sounds and sometimes a slight earache) and noted her symptoms were worse when lying down.

On the other hand, symptoms of patulous eustachian tubes tend to be worse in the upright position. A woman in this circumstance finds the sound of her own voice magnified, hollow, or echoing, and her breathing may sound like roaring in her ears. This is one woman who will actually feel better—at least in regard to these symptoms—if she catches a cold or suffers an attack of hay fever, as nasal congestion will cause the tubes to tighten up a bit.

Temporary relief of patulous tubes may also come from pinching one nostril shut, closing the mouth, and breathing in sharply through the open nostril—a maneuver most women will probably choose to reserve for a private place. Dropping the head down to chest or knees might also help, as will lying down when possible. Increased humidity can't hurt and might help. In the don't-try-this-at-home category, a review of treatments states that doctors have used "nasal douches" of boric acid and salicylic acid, injection of irritating substances into the space around the tube opening, and surgical remedies.[3] Given that none of these remedies has been thoroughly tested or even proved consistently effective, you might hesitate to seek them out, especially anything called a nasal douche. By all accounts you should avoid decongestants and diuretics, which only seem to make the symptoms worse.

Interestingly, evidence suggests that insufficient weight gain in pregnancy may in some way contribute to patulous eustachian tubes (while a larger gain does not seem to predispose a woman to eustachian tube obstruction). Other factors more prevalent in women with eustachian tube problems in pregnancy include smoking or a history of ear problems. However, eustachian tube dysfunction may occur in the absence of either factor.[4]

If you haven't complained of ear or nose problems, your particular pregnancy complaint may be stuck in your throat—literally. Like the nasopharyngeal cavity above it, the larynx can suffer tissue changes during pregnancy including swelling, dryness, and crusting. These changes may cause temporary partial or even complete loss of the voice or simply a deepening of its normal pitch. For Kim S., this has been an ongoing problem since pregnancy:

> A problem that has been very upsetting is that my voice changed during pregnancy. What upsets me is that I used to be able to sing really well. I was an alto, and after I was pregnant, I sang in a chorale group and I had to sing tenor. My voice is much deeper, and nowhere near the quality that it was. It made me sad because singing was a real joy for me. It changed, I would say, in about the sixth month of my pregnancy. I talked to my doctor about it and he said, "Well, yeah, sometimes that happens because the fluids in your body are changing. Your voice will come back." And it didn't. I mean, it has gotten better. At the end of my pregnancy I was really hoarse. I had trouble even talking. It would be really raspy.

It is also possible, though rare, to experience granulomas of the throat (as with nasal granuloma gravidarum, discussed earlier in this chapter). These merit serious treatment if they bleed or obstruct breathing, but otherwise, it is suggested that they be observed and conservatively managed because they will likely disappear shortly after delivery.

Problems with the Mouth

There may be days when you feel that being pregnant is about on par with receiving a punch in the mouth—and with good reason. Swelling of the gums is a common feature of pregnancy. In part the effect is produced by hormones. Studies have demonstrated that changes in concentrations of estrogens and progesterone cause corresponding changes in the tissue of the mouth, including the growth of new blood vessels. Couple this growth with the increased blood volume of pregnancy, and you'll understand how your gums can be at the mercy of human reproduction. Many women experience some bleeding of the gums. From this mild symptom, the scale runs all the way to significantly swollen, purplish swelling.

In this condition, your gums are hypersensitive to irritants, so dentists stress the importance of good oral hygiene to keep gum inflammation (*gingivitis*) at bay. However, since as many as 75 percent of pregnant women suffer some degree of gum inflammation, there may not be enough floss in the world to prevent it entirely. Do keep up with your dental work, and visit your dentist as soon as possible to repair any condition that might exacerbate mouth problems during the pregnancy.

Some women, perhaps 2 percent, will notice an unusual growth on their gums during pregnancy, most often appearing in the second or third month. This red or reddish purple node (or nodes—some women experience more than one) will likely bleed easily and grow quickly. It usually appears on the gums, but may occur on the tongue or other parts of the mouth, as well as on the skin. Many dentists refer to this as *pregnancy tumor*, though the use of the term is not without controversy. Some in the field of oral medicine and dentistry feel that the growth is identical to a condition (*pyogenic granuloma*) that occurs in the population at large. However, recent evidence suggests that the growth in question is unique to pregnancy and is probably influenced by placental as well as maternal hormones.[5] Since these hormones are contained in the saliva as well as the bloodstream, the gums receive a sort of double whammy that may explain the tendency of these growths to occur in the mouth.

It stands to reason that a growth promoted by pregnancy hormones would hold firm until those hormones are in retreat, and clinical experience suggests that if the growth is removed during pregnancy, recurrence is not uncommon. Current accepted practice, therefore, is not to remove these growths during the pregnancy unless they cause significant problems of some kind. After delivery, many of them disappear of their own accord. If yours does not, it's time for another trip to the dentist, since you are probably pretty tired of supporting new growth for the time being. Even fertility goddesses have to draw the line somewhere.

9

Breast Pain

THERE IS AN EARTH MOTHER SORT of notion that pregnancy somehow represents the optimal state of female functioning. This notion is by and large a crock, but there is one exception. It is fair to say that the breast is not fully formed and functional before pregnancy and truly attains its fulfillment in the gestating woman. To this fulfillment the breast responds by nearly bursting with delight. Unfortunately, all that blossoming joy can be pretty hard on the woman behind the breasts, which very quickly after conception become swollen, tender, and painful. For some women, breast sensitivity may be the first sign of pregnancy.

When you were in junior high school and desperately wanted to believe in those breast-enhancing devices, you were probably cautioned over and over again by sensible elders that the breast could not be enlarged by exercise because it is a gland. Actually, until pregnancy, the breasts are more like glands waiting to happen. Before pregnancy, the breast is largely constructed of fat and connective tissue. The underlying glandular structure is there: The beginning ducts and apparatus are laid down in fetal development, and glandular tissue develops during puberty. In pregnancy, however, the most astonishing glandular development occurs. The duct system sprouts many new branches. The *alveoli*, sacs that will contain droplets of milk, bud from the branches like flowers blooming in time-lapse photography. All this glandular structure grows right through the fat and connective tissue and actually replaces that tissue.

This tremendous development is possible because the breasts are built to receive and respond to hormonal messages throughout a woman's life, and are continuously affected by them in combination. These messages and their effects reach a peak in pregnancy.

There are three hormones known to play an active role in the development and function of the breast: estrogens, progesterone, and prolactin. These work in concert, while other hormones have "permissive roles" that allow effects of the primary three to take place. Estrogens promote growth and development of the breasts, including the ducts. In the beginning of puberty, before ovulation commences, the estrogens apparently act alone in the growth of the breasts. The development of the system of ducts and sacs, however, requires the presence of progesterone, which exerts its influence with the onset of ovulation. These roles continue cyclically throughout the reproductive years. Each month the estrogens govern a pre-ovulatory phase in which there is proliferation of the glandular cells. After ovulation, progesterone causes the dilation of the ducts and formation of secretory cells. Late in the cycle, prolactin levels increase. Together with the sexual steroids and metabolic hormones, prolactin stimulates the alveoli to begin preliminary secretory activity. Normally, however, the breasts of a nonpregnant woman will not actually secrete during this phase because the prolactin levels are not high enough.

You may have experienced all these changes in your menstrual cycle as breast fullness and tenderness, feelings compounded by increased blood flow and hormonally induced water retention in the connective tissue. Then your period arrives; the cells of the alveoli regress, and the water balloons that had been strapped to your chest magically deflate into your familiar, easy-to-live-with breasts.

With the estrogens, progesterone, and prolactin all present in raging levels during pregnancy, you get raging growth of the breasts. Enhancing this growth through permissive roles are insulin and human growth hormone, which promote cell division; cortisol, which helps the cells of the alveoli to mature into milk-producing cells; and thyroid hormones, which stimulate the increased metabolic activity of the breast. Like the sexual steroids, all these hormones are present at levels greatly increased from the prepregnancy state.

How much the breasts grow in pregnancy depends on the glandular structure laid down before pregnancy, an individual factor. It has nothing to do with the size of the breasts before pregnancy, since that is determined by fat rather than by glandular structure.

But glandular growth is not the only change accounting for the increased size of the breasts in pregnancy. Blood vessels proliferate and dilate (increase in number and size) and by term, blood flow to the breasts nearly doubles. The newly formed milk ducts also dilate, partially filling with the premilk substance called *colostrum*. The cells within the remaining connective tissue swell, and more fat is deposited under the skin. Finally, like the rest of your body, your breast tissue retains a great deal of water in pregnancy. All these factors together add an average of about three-quarters of a pound to each breast, which is something like growing a complete second set of breasts, squeezed into the same skin that already covers your preexisting pair. Because mammary temperature also increases with the increased blood flow and high metabolic rate, your breasts may feel not only swollen but hot as well.

The resulting tenderness can take a lot of the pleasure out of things you used to enjoy, such as tight hugs, as Kate remembered:

> I was three months pregnant when I saw an old friend. He gave me this big, hard hug, and it hurt so bad! I just sort of gasped out, "Not so hard!" He stepped back and said, "What are you, pregnant?" I don't know how some women manage to keep their pregnancy a secret.

Breast tenderness can also make daily routines terrifically uncomfortable, as anything that joggles the breast, from aerobic dance to running for the subway, causes pain.

Most of the breast changes begin by the third or fourth week, and the growth slows down by midpregnancy, when the production of new blood vessels and tissue cells gives way to a preparation for secretion. (If a pregnancy is terminated after sixteen weeks, the breasts will produce milk.) By late pregnancy the breasts appear to be rather insensitive to touch—a condition that will reverse dramatically when the baby is born; immediately following delivery, the nipples reach maximum sensitivity in preparation for breastfeeding.

Unlike some other pregnancy complaints such as nausea or skin rashes, the changes in the breast represent the *successful* adaptation of your body to the dramatic changes in the hormonal environment. This is one case where you don't want to "correct" or interfere with the process that is causing the symptoms. (The extremely rare exception is a case where the breasts grow literally to the size of watermelons. You can't even imagine this without seeing pictures, and you really don't want to see those pictures. This condition, called *massive hypertrophy of the breasts,* requires surgical correction.)

Your best bet is to make yourself as comfortable as possible. If your experience with brassieres has been limited to the stretchy pullover model (or less), it may be time to get acquainted with underwire. However, a bra that squeezes or compresses the breast may make you more uncomfortable, so the Wonderbra may be, as the doctors say, contraindicated. (You won't need it anyway, as you will probably have the best cleavage of your life.) The idea is to find something that minimizes the motion of the breasts when you yourself are in motion, like a sportsbra, but without too much pressure. Don't plan to shop for this bra on your lunch hour. It will probably take a lot of searching to find the right one, since you will first have to figure out your new bra size and then find the bra that fits you best.

Immersion has proved a successful therapy for excessive edema in pregnancy (see Chapter 13) and so may offer temporary relief from breast fullness and tenderness caused by water retention. You'll have to take a pretty deep bath to get your breasts immersed, but you could instead try swimming, which has the same therapeutic effect. Swimming is also a perfect choice for exercise when walking, running, or aerobic dance tend to cause more breast pain.

Even the most stoic medical writers just about break into song when they describe the lactating breast, a wondrous structure in which each cell is a perfect little model of metabolic efficiency. Your breasts are preparing themselves for the pinnacle of their career. Anyone bent on such a lofty goal is usually a little difficult to be around, often puffed up with self-importance. Be patient with your breasts. When they reach their goal, you can always say that you were behind them all the way.

10

Foot and Leg Problems

THOUGH A LOT OF THE ADVICE intended to provide comfort during pregnancy seems to include the direction "Put your feet up," many women will find the image of the little lady sitting around with her feet propped on a pile of pillows pretty much at odds with reality. The need for most people in the real world to be upright and moving for most of the day may be one reason foot problems in pregnancy are so common; but then, since there is so little chance to test the feet-up treatment, who's to say if it would really help anyway? With a foot or leg problem, as with so much else in pregnancy, probably the most helpful advice is to understand the condition and learn to cope with it–with the added instruction, as pleasing to Miss Manners as to your podiatrist, to wear the right shoes.

One of the first changes you may notice in your legs is the appearance of vascular spiders made by tiny arteries just under the skin surface that form red centers from which tinier red lines (smaller blood vessels) radiate like the legs of a spider. Similar marks on the legs appear in patients with liver disease. Since liver function in pregnancy seems largely a heroic, apparently often unsuccessful struggle by the liver to keep things running normally in the face of a tremendous hormonal overload, it seems logical that the condition of the pregnant woman's liver could predispose her to vascular spiders. Consistent with this hormonal overload theory, the predominant belief is that vascular spiders in pregnancy are caused by estrogen levels, which go so high and stay that way so long. When those levels drop after delivery, the spiders usually fade away without treatment.

Varicose veins are perhaps more common than vascular spiders and certainly more familiar (especially to those who live in resort areas where a lot of people wear shorts to the grocery store). These twisting, distended, protruding blood vessels may afflict as many as 40 percent of pregnant women. Certain symptoms associated with varicose veins, such as aching, heaviness, or tiredness in the legs, may appear in pregnancy even before the first missed period.

While the problems causing varicose veins are exacerbated by the hormones of pregnancy, the formation of varicosities depends partly on genetics. Veins in the legs have valves to keep the blood from flowing backward, but in varicose veins, incompetent valves allow blood to pool in the legs and feet. The competence of valves may be genetically determined, so a woman who is genetically predisposed to this kind of problem with blood flow stands a greater chance of developing varicose veins in pregnancy.

In some 10 percent of pregnant women with varicosities, a vein may be blocked by a blood clot, which can be a very serious condition. If you experience sudden, severe pain in your leg, along with swelling and a bluish color, call your doctor right away.

Treatment for varicose veins consists mostly of trying to encourage the blood to travel back up the legs toward the heart. One method is to attempt to compress the distended veins from the outside with the use of special elastic stockings. These may be custom-made (in which case your doctor would take the necessary measurements and order the stockings from the manufacturer), but even advocates of the custom variety admit that women may find it more practical to purchase over-the-counter brands that are readily available and less expensive.[1] There is also the no-expense treatment of elevating the legs whenever possible. This prescription often includes advice to sleep with the legs on pillows, but ask your doctor; at least one author writes that sleeping with pillows behind the legs may *increase* the risk of a blood clot.[2]

Both vascular spiders and varicose veins are representative of the changes pregnancy works upon the circulatory system. As the farthest outposts of that system, your feet and legs are sensitive to any changes in the efficiency or stability of the blood vessels. Such changes are thought to be responsible for the appearance in some pregnant women of *cutis marmorata*, a condition in which the extremities take on a mottled, reddish blue discoloration when exposed to cold. It may look strange, but it is probably no cause for alarm and will likely resolve after delivery. Meanwhile, keep your feet warm.

In pregnancy, red blood cells may be forced through the walls of newly fragile, unusually permeable blood vessels into the surrounding tissue. When this happens with the blood vessels of the skin, the result may be purplish spots, which tend to appear on the legs or feet around the beginning of the second trimester. No treatment is suggested in the current literature, since, like many skin changes related to circulatory function, they tend to resolve quickly after delivery.

Of course, as your pregnancy advances, you'll be seeing less and less of your feet anyway, and concern over their more colorful changes may give way to problems that you feel more than see. With hormones, weight gain, and fluid retention working together, most women do eventually feel the influences of pregnancy in their lower extremities.

Common complaints in pregnancy include foot and leg pain and fatigue. Many women share the complaint Dawn T. voiced in her seventh month: "My feet hurt as if I have been on them for eighteen hours when I have hardly been on them at all." Research on such complaints is scanty, but there seem to be at least some sound theories to explain how the foot is altered by pregnancy.

In nonpregnant circumstances, the architecture of the foot holds up pretty well under a considerable amount of strain. Because the foot is a well-organized collection of twenty-six bones (held together with *ligaments*, bands of tough tissue) instead of a solid peg, there is room for adjustment for all sorts of positions and activities. Pregnancy calls for new adjustments, especially to weight gain. A body doesn't just take on thirty to sixty pounds in a few months' time without its placing some demands on the feet, particularly when much of that weight is in one spot. As the body's center of gravity moves toward the front, the pregnant woman walks at an unaccustomed angle, resulting in strain to the feet and legs.

Even before weight gain begins, the foot changes. The hormone *relaxin*, produced in pregnancy to relax the ligaments holding pelvic bones together, likely has both an indirect and a direct effect on the feet. The indirect effect occurs when the relaxing of the pelvic and surrounding joints changes the way a woman stands and walks (even before any appreciable weight gain, as relaxin is at its peak in the first trimester). At this time the posture of the feet is also changed and may produce pain in the back, knees, or thighs as well as in the feet. Relaxin may also act directly on the ligaments of the foot. Studies have found that pregnant women tend to have a significantly increased range of motion in many of the joints of the foot.[3] It seems logical that the effects of relaxin are not limited to the ligaments of the pelvis and that a large ligament of the foot, the *plantar calcaneonavicular* ligament, could be similarly affected. This ligament is suspected as a target for relaxin because, unlike other ligaments of the foot, it contains much of the same elastic fiber found in the pelvic ligaments. (Though relaxin's specific actions are not yet fully understood, research has demonstrated the hormone's ability to break down this particular type of fiber.) Further, if the plantar ligament were thus stretched and loosened by relaxin, the result (particularly the tendency to roll the weight outward to the sides of the feet) could be the type of "foot fault" to which much of foot and leg pain can logically be attributed.

With the idea that such inappropriate motion is the primary evil, podiatrists recommend shoes that will support the feet and prevent improper motion as much as possible. Remembering that your foot size is probably larger in pregnancy, choose shoes both long and wide enough for your toes to move around in. Arch support is very important. Athletic shoes are often helpful in this regard, and wearing shoes with their shock-absorbing properties is recommended in pregnancy. Podiatrists also suggest wearing shoes that reduce heel motion (like running shoes with soles that extend backward behind the heels), so it's time to store the spike heels for a while. However, if you are used to wearing only high heels and suddenly switch to flats, you may experience some pain in the back of the legs as a result of the strain from the sudden adjustment. Again, you would do better to switch to athletic shoes with lots of support than to slip into ballerina flats.

Pregnancy's effects on the spine (see Chapter 11) can also produce leg pain ranging from mild to nearly incapacitating. Of her first pregnancy, Kim D. said:

> The leg pain started at about seven months along. It was like hitting your funny bone, but it would shoot down my leg, starting about from the hip bone and "shocking" all the way down to my heel. The ache seemed to rest there in my heel for a minute or two, almost like a bruise. I would get a few shocks a week, and only two were so bad that my knee gave out (as if someone snuck up behind me and pushed my knee in to make me lose balance). Thank goodness I wasn't walking or climbing stairs at the time! I grabbed the wall divider and didn't fall. My doctor explained it off as "normal" and something vague like "the baby must be bumping a nerve." I took his word for it and just coped with it.

In Kim's next pregnancy, she had the same problem, and this time her doctor took more notice:

> The "zings" were stronger and more frequent. I described them to my doctor "as if my leg is popping out of the socket." The whole hip would almost audibly pop or creak, and then I would get that shock down my leg. At thirty-two weeks my doctor witnessed me getting off the examining table and my knee giving way and put me on immediate maternity leave. This time, my OB said that my body was making room for the delivery and my hips were actually moving themselves out of the way. (Great—bigger hips!)

The "shocks" Kim felt and the inability to support weight strongly suggest a nerve problem. Chiropractors and physical therapists are trained to diagnose these problems by simple muscle testing (not requiring machines) that can determine which nerve is at fault. If you experience these kinds of leg problems in pregnancy, you may obtain some relief from physical therapy or chiropractic manipulation.

A virtually universal complaint of pregnancy is increased foot size. Many women move to larger shoe sizes in pregnancy, and some never go back. "Oh, my feet grew," said Colleen. "Big time. I had to buy new shoes. I'm an eight now and I was a seven." Colleen said that about eighteen months after her daughter's birth, she was able to wear some seven and a halfs, but they felt tight. Anna agreed, saying that almost two years after her son was born, "some shoes still fit OK and others don't."

The spreading of bones described earlier in this chapter has long been suspected as one reason for such changes in shoe size. However, one team of researchers measured the length and width of subjects' feet at thirteen weeks and thirty-five weeks of gestation as well as eight weeks postpartum and found no significant changes. (They do note that changes might have taken place before the thirteenth week, as relaxin is at a high level early in pregnancy.) On the other hand, measurements of *volume*—the bulk of the foot—were much increased between thirteen and thirty-five weeks, and the volume postpartum remained higher than at thirteen weeks. Apparently, the feet were simply holding more of something in roughly the same amount of bone space, which would account for the swollen feeling most subjects described.[4]

The researchers speculate that much of the increased volume must be caused by deposits of fat in the feet. If fluid retention were the sole culprit, they note, then the feet should quickly return to their prepregnancy volume after delivery, since fluid loss is usually rapid postpartum. Instead, the volume of the feet remains larger, suggesting the presence of more soft tissue—in other words, fat.

If these researchers are right, there appears to be little anyone can do about increased foot size. During pregnancy, doctors counsel against the use of diuretics (water-reducing medications) for swelling of the feet and legs. As for added fat, unless someone develops some surefire foot-slimming exercises (a new opportunity for entrepreneurs?), we must pretty much learn to live with it. Try to look on the bright side. I have a friend with disproportionately small feet who says she falls down a lot. As a mother, you will need stability and balance in all aspects of life, including feet that will hold you up. Just remember to add a *W* after your shoe size, and you will stride through motherhood with ease.

11

Backache

THE FACT THAT MANY AILMENTS ARE an almost inescapable part of pregnancy does not make them any easier to live with, but it may make them easier for your doctor to dismiss. A recent discussion of pregnancy-related backache notes that "women are often told simply to accept back pain as an expected burden of pregnancy."[1] Being pregnant may set you up for a lot of this sort of counseling. (Two physicians from Baylor Medical School actually began their discussion of a pregnancy-related skin condition with a quote from Genesis: "I will greatly increase the pangs of your childbearing; in pain shall you bring forth children."[2]) Burdens, it seems, are to be stoically shouldered as the moral and medical lot of pregnant women—and in the presence of any burden, it is the spine that does the bearing.

In the last weeks of her pregnancy, Dawn T. wrote:

> At about thirty-four weeks, I pulled a muscle in my lower back on the left side while vacuuming. It's been a week and a half since then, and it is not any better. Sitting is most comfortable, walking is rough, and up and down stairs is excruciating. Lying down isn't too bad if I can stay in the right position. If not, I wake up with the muscle in a spasm. I've been having false contractions off and on for four days, and they intensify the pain in my back. This has had a large effect on my life. I'm not cooking or cleaning, and small tasks have become things to dread. (Putting a load of laundry in, which involves stairs and carrying, for instance.) Getting in and out of the car is very painful, so I go only where I have to. I am also a little concerned about going through labor with my back already hurting so much.

There is a Saturday morning image that comes to mind when you consider the spine: a cartoon character running from point A to point B with a stack of plates shifting and teetering in his hands. The vertebrae of the spine are stacked a bit like those plates, though under ideal circumstances there is considerably less shifting. Still, though people use "spine" and "backbone" to describe an unyielding nature, the makeup of the spine provides not rigidity, but flexibility and a wide range of movement for the human body.

The thirty-three vertebrae are not stacked in a straight, rigid column, which would offer little flexibility or resilience. Instead, the stack curves toward the front of the body at the neck (cervical vertebrae), backward through the shoulder and rib region (thoracic vertebrae), then forward again in the lower back (lumbar vertebrae). The *sacrum* and *coccyx*, both composed of a number of fused vertebrae, curve backward once more at the bottom of the spine. The primary joint between each two vertebrae is the *intervertebral disc*, made of thick cartilage that allows some range of movement while keeping the arrangement, position, and length of the total spine more or less consistent.

This arrangement is built to take some punishment. It absorbs shock, supports the whole skeleton, bears the body's weight, and resists, as much as possible, the compressive force of the universe. Because that force becomes greater as it travels down the spine, the lower vertebral bodies bear the brunt of gravity. To compensate, the lumbar vertebrae are the largest vertebrae of the spine; still, the load and the curvature combined make this region the most prone to problems like disc herniations, when the intervertebral disc is forced outward from its normal position. Finally, the weight of the world comes to rest on the sacrum, which resembles the keystone of an arch[3]—an arch whose stability relies on its only fixed points, the (normally) rigid union of the sacroiliac joints, where the bones of the spine finally meet the bones of the hips.

All this information applies to the spine under normal conditions—that is, to people who are not walking around with ten-pound watermelons strapped to their abdomens. But as pregnancy rearranges your life, so it rearranges your insides, presenting your vertebral column with a lot of new challenges. As early as twelve weeks, the uterus is already shoving other organs aside. With the uterus moving forward and the intestines edging up and outward, the body's center of gravity moves up, forward, and sideways all at once. Your spine, bearer of all burdens, adapts as best it can—though not always with heroic silence.

Ann H. wrote:

> As I got close to term, I got such a horrible backache, low down, like a knife in the buttocks really. I could barely walk. I couldn't believe how much it hurt, that anyone could actually live like this.

> I couldn't walk from one end of the kitchen to the other without terrible, terrible pain. Labor was a snap compared to those three weeks. I remember thinking as I went to the OB for appointments, having to cross an enormous parking lot with my active two-year-old in tow, that I needed a disabled sticker for my car so I could park in a handicapped spot for a week or two!

Exactly how the spine adjusts is a matter of some dispute. Most people think pregnant women have a swaybacked stance. In the medical world, this image has translated into a common belief that pregnancy exaggerates the forward curve of the lumbar region. However, as early as 1943, some lone voices in the medical establishment have argued that the spine compensates for the new center of gravity with a *backward* motion.[4] The whole vertebral column moves to the rear, a movement that may actually flatten the lumbar curve. When a region of the spine loses its vital curvature, trouble is almost guaranteed to follow.

At the same time, the spine's support systems dwindle. Normally, the load on the lumbar region is counterbalanced by the force provided by muscles and ligaments. Both are compromised by pregnancy.

The abdominal muscles are particularly weak. A study of abdominal muscle performance in pregnant and nonpregnant women led to the hardly surprising discovery that in late pregnancy, most of the subjects could not perform a basic sit-up (hands behind the head, knees flexed, soles of feet on table). Actually, the researchers found that few of their pregnant subjects could even rise from the examining table without help, let alone perform a sit-up. Their conclusion is that the extreme stretching of the abdominal wall causes a muscular insufficiency, leaving these muscles unable to provide the necessary balance for the strained muscles around the spine.[5]

Meanwhile, the ligaments that should be holding the whole business together may be showing the influence of relaxin, a hormone that during pregnancy increases to ten times the nonpregnant level. Relaxin softens connective tissue; its primary target is the *symphysis pubis*, the joint between the pubic bones. It also affects the sacroiliac joints, causing looseness in the hips.

Thus a predisposition toward back pain does seem to be an almost inescapable feature of pregnancy. Still, it is only a predisposition and not a certainty. The true incidence is unknown because back pain, like almost every other nonthreatening complaint of pregnancy, is not well researched. The wide range reported in existing studies (in which from 48 to 90 percent of subjects report some back pain) suggests that methods and measurements have not been terribly consistent. However, few studies have found the incidence to be lower than 48 percent. Of all subjects with backache, the number reporting severe or disabling pain runs from about 10 to 30 percent.

If every pregnant body undergoes the same biomechanical changes, why doesn't every woman suffer backache in pregnancy? Research has turned up no firm answers and only a few suggestions. Studies conflict on whether age and number of deliveries are related to back pain, but they generally agree that the amount of weight gained during pregnancy does *not* have a direct influence on whether the mother will develop back pain. Also apparently unrelated to pain are the mother's weight before pregnancy and the weight of the baby with one small exception: One study found a slight suggestion that among the women with back pain, those developing pain in the third trimester tended to be carrying heavier babies.[6]

This suggestion, these study authors note, brings up the possibility that there are different types of pregnancy backaches, some of them related to factors in particular trimesters. For instance, some women report backache in the first trimester, long before the development of any excess load on the spine. Perhaps these women are particularly sensitive to the effects of relaxin, which may already be present in high levels in the early weeks of pregnancy. Meanwhile, women suffering third-trimester backache may be feeling the effects of heavier babies or weakened abdominal muscles.

The fact that some women suffer backache largely or exclusively at night suggests still other factors may be at work–perhaps a problem with circulation in the lumbar region, which is compromised by the enlarged uterus when the pregnant woman is lying on her back (see Chapter 5). This is just one example of how the nervous and musculoskeletal systems may be effected by other body systems, effects resulting in pain.

Emotions, too, may play a role. The lumbar region often becomes the seat of tension during times of emotional stress, when the muscles of the lower back tend to suffer excessive contraction. The resulting strain can produce muscle spasms which are not only quite painful themselves but can lead to other problems. Further, the continuous tension tires the muscles, which makes it all the more difficult to maintain correct posture and so increases the likelihood of back pain.[7]

All these theories focus on the lumbar discs, but research suggests that there may be more than one problem in more than one region. Some researchers have questioned whether back pain in pregnancy is more likely caused by problems with a lumbar disc or with the sacroiliac joint. The symptoms can be hard to distinguish, as the supposedly "characteristic" radiating leg pain of lumbar disc disease can also be produced by sacroiliac problems, as well as by severe muscle spasms. In various papers, doctors have attempted to prove or disprove that women in general are predisposed to lumbar disc disease and that pregnancy increases the predisposition. According to one review, one study found 39 percent of subjects developed lumbar disc symptoms during pregnancy, while another found only five pregnant women with evidence of herniated lumbar discs among 48,760 patients.[8] Given this huge discrepancy and the fact that the review author complained about lax research methods in both studies, it seems that there is little reliable evidence in either direction.

What's more, a disc does not have to be herniated to produce pain. Discs themselves can hurt, through nerve endings in the outer cover of the disc. If inflammatory cells penetrate this outer cover, the stimulated nerve endings may signal pain.[9]

The possibility of sacroiliac problems is, if anything, more controversial than lumbar disc theories, with some authors arguing loudly in favor of a sacroiliac syndrome while others vehemently denying that such a syndrome even exists. However, muscle testing can distinguish sacroiliac dysfunction from other problems, and studies making use of such testing have indeed found a significant prevalence of sacroiliac problems in pregnant women with back pain. Data also suggest that a diagnosis of sacroiliac dysfunction carries a prognosis for a slow recovery. In one study, patients with sacroiliac problems (two-thirds of the study's seventy-nine subjects) had back pain of longer duration, with most suffering symptoms several months postpartum.[10]

Proper treatment focused on the affected area may improve this prognosis. One OB noted that over the course of 15 years, he had successfully treated hundreds of cases of pregnancy backache with a simple manipulation of the sacroiliac joints—a procedure he described in detail, with photographs, in a 1958 OB-GYN journal.[11] Over the years, research has continued to confirm his experience. Most recently, in a 1991 study pregnant subjects who were diagnosed with sacroiliac dysfunction were treated with rotational manipulation of the sacroiliac joints. Ten of the eleven women experienced relief from their pain and showed no further signs of the sacroiliac problem.[12]

Whatever the region, whatever the cause or combination of causes, here's a short list of activities that studies have found tend to increase pain: standing, sitting, walking, bending, lifting, twisting, coughing, sneezing, straining during a bowel movement; also heavy work, seated work, disliking your job, being tired from your job at the end of the day, and being unable to take breaks while on the job. As noted earlier, a substantial number of women also experience pain when lying down.

Evidently, then, you should not plan on preventing backache by avoiding activities that may produce it, since it is pretty hard to get through a day without standing, sitting, walking, or lying down, even if you could quit your job and stifle the occasional cough or sneeze. However, there are positive actions you might take that have helped some other women.

Feeling Better

Posture. Your first line of defense is a firm—and correct—stance. If you have been experiencing back problems, you are no doubt heartily sick of this advice already, and it is probably true that simple posture awareness is more effective in preventing mild pain or fatigue of the lower back than in relieving really severe symptoms. Even in severe cases, however, you must start with correct posture before other pain relief mechanisms can do their work. Try to maintain a "neutral lumbar lordosis"[13]—that is, while avoiding a swayback posture with the weight of the abdomen thrust forward, you should not overcompensate by trying to flatten the lumbar curve. Wearing high-heeled shoes causes the sacrum to tilt downward, exaggerating the lumbar curve, so stow your girl shoes for the duration of the pregnancy. When standing or sitting for a long time, try placing one foot on a low stool to avoid the strain caused by a continuous downward drag on the pelvis. In low seats—particularly in automobiles—it may be helpful to use a lower-back support cushion.[14]

Exercise. In conjunction with posture awareness, probably the most common prescription for back pain is exercise. Unfortunately, the types of exercises usually prescribed may not be particularly helpful to pregnant women. For example, for nonpregnant patients many physicians recommend sit-ups to improve abdominal muscle tone. As noted earlier, however, by late pregnancy sit-ups are difficult or impossible. Further, data are inconsistent on whether regular exercise actually prevents back pain for pregnant women. In one study women who performed aerobic exercise at least twice a week for at least twenty minutes each time had significantly fewer complaints of lower back pain.[15] However, another study offered no such result. In this study, nonpregnant subjects who engaged in four or more hours of exercise per week did indeed have less back pain, but that same level of exercise in pregnant women did not protect against pain and possibly even created a predisposition toward it.[16] The differing levels of exercise may have been a factor; twice a week for twenty minutes is a lot less than four or more hours per week. It is apparently important that pregnant women carefully choose nonstrenuous exercises and pursue them only to a level of comfort. (See Appendix for more recommendations on exercise.)

A widely prescribed lower-back exercise for pregnant women involves pelvic lifts. To perform this exercise, lie on your back with legs comfortably apart and bent at the knees, soles of the feet flat on the floor. Press your lower back flat against the floor. (It may help to imagine pulling your abdomen in to touch your spine.) Release (allowing the back to assume its natural curve), then press again. This is actually only the first half of the exercise, but it may be as far as you can get;

even so, it is worth performing regularly, both to strengthen abdominal muscles and to develop the habit of proper pelvic positioning when standing or sitting. The second step, for those who are able to perform it, offers additional strengthening of abdominal and gluteal (rear end) muscles. From the spine-against-the-floor position, squeeze your buttocks together and attempt to lift your bottom slightly while keeping the lumbar region in contact with the floor. Just the slightest lift is possible before the spine starts to come up too, so don't push it; your focus is more on tightening the muscles of the buttocks than achieving any height. Release and repeat a few times, never exceeding the point of comfort.[17]

From this same position, you can try a few other exercises. You can do a small sit-up, just raising your head and shoulders to form about a 30 degree angle with the floor, holding, and releasing. You can stretch your hamstrings (tight hamstrings are a source of lower back strain) by gently extending and raising first one leg and then the other, no higher than a 90 degree angle with the floor (straight up and down—but don't force your leg this high if you experience pain). You can also try slowly bringing alternate knees and then both knees at once toward the chest, but it is hard to imagine how this maneuver might be accomplished beyond about five months.[18]

Although data regarding aerobic exercise as a preventative measure are inconclusive, some women find that getting into motion offers some short-term relief of backache. Swimming is an excellent choice, as it allows motion and exercise without the stress of weight load. Because immersion has also been demonstrated to dramatically relieve fluid retention of pregnancy (see Chapter 13), swimming may offer added benefits by relieving the pressure of fluid retained in the tissues around the spine. Stationary biking, while it does not offer the all-around benefits of swimming, is another good choice for exercise that does not jar the spine.

Walking is also a standard prescription, though it is perhaps not the universal relief mechanism some health care providers believe it to be. Walking may have more to offer as a preventative measure with cumulative benefits than as an immediate pain reliever—and of course, it has to be done with correct posture. In one study, subjects voted walking the least effective of eight popular measures against backache.[19] Still, the fact that it was listed at all signifies that some women have found it useful, and it certainly can't hurt.

Among the measures that women reported more effective than walking were position changes (from standing or sitting to lying, from lying to standing, from standing to sitting), pain-relief medications, and hot water baths. Both hot water bottles and ice have been suggested for application to the small of the back; women have reported success with both.

Intervention. When intervention for back pain seems necessary, it makes sense to choose a professional who can focus on your spine instead of your uterus. That means your first choice may not be your obstetrician, but a chiropractor or physical therapist. Studies show that patients with lower back pain are more satisfied with the care they receive from these professionals than from medical doctors.[20]

Chiropractic, like any field, has its praiseworthy professionals and its bottom dwellers. It is vital that you distinguish among them. Ask your friends for recommendations, and consider those names in light of some "guidelines for identifying a competent chiropractor" provided in a collaborative article by a family physician and a chiropractor.[21] According to these doctors, a chiropractor should focus mainly on musculoskeletal disorders, which he or she treats with manipulative techniques (manual adjustments). A good chiropractor does not need to perform routine X rays, as much of his or her diagnosis can be accomplished with simple muscle testing, without the aid of machines. Look out for chiropractors who seem to prescribe extended treatment for every patient, as many problems can be resolved quickly. Also avoid anyone charging a lump sum up front for a proposed course of treatment. Look for a chiropractor who has graduated from a school accredited by the Council on Chiropractic Education. Finally, as a professional, your chiropractor should be willing to allow your physician to observe your treatment, should you desire.

Medical treatments. Back pain, like other complaints, may force a pregnant woman to consider the difficult question of appropriate medication. Exactly what medicine might best serve any back patient, let alone a pregnant one, is still uncertain. Many medications are simply ineffective for pain involving compromised nerves.[22] However, it is possible to have some influence over pain with medications that inhibit the synthesis of *prostaglandins*, substances that are secreted during the inflammatory process. Prostaglandins do not directly produce pain but make the body more sensitive to it. Over-the-counter drugs that inhibit prostaglandins include aspirin and ibuprofen (Motrin, Advil). Discuss these with your doctor before taking them in pregnancy. Most physicians are more likely to recommend acetaminophen, which unfortunately does not have the same action. Still, it may provide some relief, and it is by far the most widely recommended pain medication for pregnancy.

A process called *transcutaneous electrical nerve stimulation* (TENS) has been used to treat lower-back pain. This process involves the application (through electrodes on the skin) of tiny electrical impulses to nerve endings in the painful area. The theory is that these electrical shocks block pain signals by giving the nerve endings something else to feel. However, over the years little evidence has accumulated to demonstrate that this technique really helps anybody.

A more invasive procedure, the injection of corticosteroids directly into the lumbar region, has likewise not shown significant results and carries considerable risks even for nonpregnant patients. One study found this treatment inferior to the use of a pain-relief spray (vapocoolant) in conjunction with stretching exercises.[23]

A noninvasive treatment that has helped some women with pregnancy back pain is the use of a special device called a *trochanteric belt* that is worn to minimize movement in the pelvic region. Particularly if your backache develops early in pregnancy—suggesting that looseness in the joints caused by relaxin may be to blame—you may want to discuss the use of such a device with your care provider.

Anyone treating or living with back pain in pregnancy should also be prepared to deal with potential emotional effects. Research suggests that only a small percentage of nerve fibers transmit pain signals directly along "pain pathways" to the appropriate areas of the brain. A whopping 85 percent transmit their messages through brain areas affecting behavior, emotions, and the workings of internal organs.[24] If pain continues for long periods, emotional responses such as anxiety and depression are all but inevitable—and only exacerbated by pregnancy, which can wreak havoc on the emotions through so many pathways. Recognizing the likelihood of such responses may help you, your family, and your care provider to deal with them with a minimum of friction and misplaced blame.

It is difficult to predict when pregnancy-related back pain may resolve. Factors such as laxity of the ligaments and weakness of the abdominal muscles can persist for several months postpartum. At the same time, you will be taxing your back with a lot of stooping and lifting as you care for your baby. One study reports the not-very-heartening finding that back pain usually resolved within six months after delivery but that women with back pain in previous pregnancies suffered symptoms longer; 82 percent still reported pain after eighteen months.[25] These figures only emphasize the importance of developing and maintaining a good back-care regimen during pregnancy. The measure of strength and tone provided by exercises conscientiously performed throughout pregnancy may shorten recovery time after delivery. If pain persists, it helps to have already established a relationship with a specialist who can continue a course of treatment based on what he or she has already learned about your body. Back pain, like pregnancy, is a process of adaptations to a changing internal environment. Find someone who can adapt your treatment in sync with your body, and eventually the process will end in relief.

12

Carpal Tunnel Syndrome

CARPAL TUNNEL SYNDROME, A TROUBLING and sometimes disabling condition involving pain, numbness, and weakness of the hands, is getting a lot of press these days as an occupational hazard. Among the occupations that carry this risk are typing, assembly line work, and gestating a human being. The literature of obstetrics states that pregnancy-related carpal tunnel syndrome and a more generalized but similar ailment called *hand syndrome of pregnancy* (HSP) are common, though the reported incidence varies wildly, from 1 to 50 percent of all pregnancies.

Sufferers of carpal tunnel syndrome and HSP describe a progression beginning with tingling and numbness in the hands. This tingling gradually becomes more painful and may develop into cramping, spasmodic pain accompanied by weakness that causes some women difficulty in normal activities such as writing or holding objects. The fingers feel stiff and swollen (sometimes swelling is actually visible). Studies suggest it is common for women to experience more severe symptoms in the dominant hand (that is, in the right hand for right-handed women, the left for left-handed women). However, both hands are usually affected to some degree. In cases of HSP, symptoms may also include an ache or a feeling of tiredness or heaviness in the arms.

"I had horrible carpal tunnel," wrote Welmoed. "Couldn't move my hands at all for at least the first hour or two of each day." Christy also remembered a disabling bout: "Toward the end of my pregnancy, my wrist started hurting so badly. I had already done my thank-you notes, and I was so glad because by the end I couldn't write anything. It was so painful."

Carpal tunnel syndrome is distinguished from HSP by the specific sites of the numbness, tingling, and pain: the thumb, the index and middle fingers, and sometimes one side of the ring finger. These are the areas whose nerve impulses come from the median nerve, which passes through the carpal tunnel, a fibrous trough leading from the forearm to the palm of the hand. The "roof" of this trough is the transverse carpal ligament, a thick band of tissue that runs crossways at the bottom of the hand. The thickness of this ligament and the fibrous walls of the trough make the dimensions of the carpal tunnel nonnegotiable. This unyielding nature presents a problem when some condition (including a misaligned wrist fracture, tumors, or tissue swelling from injury or infection) causes a change in the volume of the tunnel's contents. The slightest tightness within the channel compresses the median nerve, which provides both sensory and motor impulses to the fingers noted above.

On examination, a patient suffering carpal tunnel syndrome will demonstrate impairment of median nerve function with specific physical signs, including tenderness of the wrist when the median nerve area is pressed, tingling and numbness produced by tapping the same area, and worsened symptoms when the wrist is stretched or flexed. A readout of electrical impulses will show that the signals from the median nerve are definitely slowed.

There is little argument, then, that the symptoms of carpal tunnel syndrome relate to problems with the median nerve. The question of exactly what causes the nerve compression or irritation is not so satisfactorily answered and has generated a number of theories. When you toss in HSP, in which symptoms affect all the fingers or even the arms, a few more theories bubble to the surface.

Probably the most commonly accepted explanation for carpal tunnel syndrome in pregnancy is that fluid retention causes excessive pressure within the tunnel and compresses the median nerve. Fluid retention is certainly an obvious culprit, since every pregnant woman experiences it to some degree and the connection to carpal tunnel pressure is eminently logical. In one study of carpal tunnel syndrome in pregnancy, all subjects had experienced swelling of the hands to the point of being unable to wear their usual rings, and an unusually high percentage of subjects had suffered preeclampsia (a high blood pressure condition that involves fluid retention).[1] However, several other studies have noted very little edema (the swelling characteristic of excess fluid retention) and no preeclampsia in study subjects. Further, though most studies associate carpal tunnel with the third trimester, at least one states that symptoms have been reported and median nerve delay confirmed with readouts of electrical activity as early as the third month, when no noticeable edema is present.[2] Finally, the fact that the syndrome in some cases persists after delivery (and in extreme cases is relieved only by surgery) suggests that, at least in some women, factors other than fluid retention may play a role.

Other facts suggest that the condition may be hormonally influenced. For one thing, it is simply much more common in women, who suffer the syndrome about five times more often than men. It has also been associated with oral contraceptive use, and sometimes appears in breastfeeding mothers. Of course, it is the hormones of pregnancy that instruct the body to retain fluid, so edema and hormones are not mutually exclusive as precipitating factors. However, hormones may come into play in other ways. For example, relaxin, the hormone that allows loosening of the pelvis in pregnancy, may also affect the ligaments of the hand and wrist in some way that predisposes to carpal tunnel syndrome. Relaxation of these ligaments might allow more fluid to accumulate in the tunnel. Or perhaps the tightness of the tunnel is caused not so much by increased contents as by decreased size. Perhaps the pregnancy hormones, which stimulate growth of new blood vessels and tissue, cause thickening of the tissue of the tunnel walls. Still another theory holds that changes in the nerve tissue spread along the nerves, causing them to become inelastic, so that stretching them produces pain.[3] This theory would explain not only carpal tunnel syndrome but HSP, since it allows for involvement of the nerves over a larger area. However, the changes in the nerve tissue are as yet only theoretical.

Also mediated by hormones are the many metabolic changes of pregnancy, and in at least one study doctors looked for signs of disturbed calcium metabolism as a possible explanation of carpal tunnel. Since calcium regulates nerve-to-muscle communication, a lack of adequate calcium may impair conduction of nerve impulses. However, no subject in this study showed any signs of hypocalcemia.[4]

Other doctors believe that carpal tunnel and HSP involve less body chemistry than body mechanics. If the forward curve of the spine in pregnancy is particularly pronounced, and if that curve is coupled with a forward slump of the neck and shoulders, the combination causes drag and tension on two major nerves—the median (which would explain the symptoms of carpal tunnel) and the ulnar (which would account for the more diffuse symptoms of HSP). However, these postural changes do not occur until the third trimester; thus the theory fails to account for any symptoms occurring earlier in the pregnancy.[5]

All of these theories were developed around the 1960s, some fifteen to twenty years after an association between carpal tunnel syndrome and pregnancy was first noted in the literature. As the syndrome gained more recognition, doctors sought an explanation in order to determine the appropriate treatment. Those who subscribed to the "edema in the tunnel" theory prescribed diuretics to reduce fluid retention, with mixed and inconclusive results. Those who ascribed the symptoms to postural problems claimed a good cure rate with posture awareness and exercises.

Other suggested treatments were based more on relieving the symptoms than on correcting the cause. One such nonspecific treatment, injections of hydrocortisone into the carpal tunnel (to reduce inflammation), has proved largely unsuccessful. Some papers mention the (unsuccessful) use of sedatives; presumably the prescribing doctors were of the infuriating crowd noted in one paper who wrote the syndrome off as an "attention-getting mechanism."[6]

In most of the studies, subjects seem to have attained the most relief by wearing a splint, mostly at night, to hold the wrist in a position that did not stretch or irritate the median nerve. This noninvasive treatment is a good choice for a pregnancy-related condition. Some women also reported temporary relief by hanging their hands over the sides of the bed, which certainly seems worth a try.

Many women have obtained excellent results from chiropractic adjustment. The cervical disc problems described earlier are exactly the sort of mechanical disturbance that chiropractors are trained to address. If you have never visited a chiropractor, it's a good idea to ask around for recommendations. You may also consider the guidelines for finding a chiropractor in Chapter 11.

In most cases, hand and arm symptoms clear up quickly after delivery, usually within a month or two. This was the case for Christy, who said that her carpal tunnel "went away on its own. It took about two months to go away." However, she noted that two years after the birth of her son, "my wrist is still real prone, after a lot of repetitive things, to get real sore." Like Christy, you may find that some trace of pain and numbness lingers on. If your symptoms seem endlessly persistent and disabling, report the problem to your doctor. You may wish to try the whole range of treatments available. Some women, with symptoms persisting as long as twenty months after delivery, have found relief only with surgical intervention. Remember, though, that the syndrome has also been associated with breastfeeding (though usually not in women who experienced it while pregnant). You may wish to delay any decisions about surgery until after weaning, to see if the symptoms resolve at that time.

13

Edema

Every organism is made up of cells, and cells contain so much water—60 to 65 percent of their makeup—that it's a wonder the world isn't awash with sloshing sounds as all of us organisms go about our daily business. It has been suggested that since our bodies contain so much water, our souls must be floating around inside us on rubber life rafts. If that is true, the soul might be in danger of drowning during pregnancy, when a woman accumulates an average of six to eight liters of additional fluid. However, the raftbound spirit is hardly in for a whitewater trip. This accumulated fluid does not rush through the body like a flood, but slows, pools, sits. In normal pregnancy, blood volume increases about 50 percent, but blood pressure actually drops, leaving an awful lot of blood that is in no hurry to get anywhere. Further, the increased blood volume accounts for only some of the fluid gain of pregnancy. Much of the rest is fluid collected in the tissue outside the blood vessels, where it produces effects for the amusement of your friends and family, who may find ghoulish fascination in poking fingers into your feet to watch them pit.

Edema, the presence of excess fluid in body tissues, is the subject of much study and aggressive treatment when it occurs in nonpregnant people, as in cases of heart or kidney disease. However, as an almost universal complaint of pregnancy, it is almost universally ignored in obstetrical texts, which generally have little to say about any condition that does not connote disease or disorder in pregnancy, no matter how common or how unpleasant. True to form, the medical books do discuss certain cases of edema as symptomatic of possible hypertensive disease (*eclampsia*). Nevertheless, despite this association, edema is by no means always evidence of a threatening condition. After all, you are adding eight liters of fluid to your system. Think about that in terms of Pepsi bottles, and you'll realize there's a lot of extra fluid that has to be stored somewhere.

How and why does the body retain so much fluid in pregnancy? There are a couple of reigning assumptions regarding the *how*, but the *why* seems still to be anyone's guess.

Fluid balance in the body is normally accomplished by the kidneys, where blood is filtered through clusters of capillaries called *glomeruli*, which remove water, salts, and waste products from the blood. These substances eventually pass through the renal tubules, where most of the water and salt is reabsorbed into the blood before the rest passes out of the body in the urine.

In pregnancy, the filtration rate in the glomeruli is increased 50 percent or more, a condition appearing to favor sodium depletion. Yet the absorption of water and salt from the renal tubules is also increased. More water and salt filtered out, more water and salt back in; the result is increased volume of blood *plasma* (the fluid component of blood), with increased sodium content to maintain the proper balance of electrolytes.

At the same time, decreased resistance in blood vessels leads to higher filtration of fluid through capillaries into the surrounding tissue. In the tiny capillaries, with their very thin walls, blood comes into its closest contact with body tissues. Oxygen and nutrients are released from the blood into the tissues, passing through the thin walls of the capillaries. In exchange, waste products from the tissues pass into the blood, to be carried into veins and ultimately back to the heart.

To maintain the constant exchange of substances in and out of the tissues, blood flow to the capillaries must remain constant even as the heart alternately pumps and relaxes. To maintain flow while the heart is resting between beats, the muscular walls of the arteries contract after each beat. If this reflexive constriction is impaired, as it is in pregnancy by the lower resistance of the vessels, blood can pool in the capillaries. The resulting increase in hydrostatic pressure causes overfiltration of the blood from the capillaries, so that more water flows into the tissues.

The swelling may be visible anywhere. "My nose spread across my face," groaned Colleen. "I mean, it hurt to smile." Remembering that her eyesight seemed less acute, Colleen speculated that facial swelling even caused her eyeballs to be forced out of shape. "You know, when I smiled, my eyes probably went like *this*," she said, stretching them into slits. "I was, *walla walla walla walla*, full of water! My *Birkenstocks* didn't even fit. I had them loosened up. I thought I had elephantiasis."

Anna said that she, too, had marked edema toward the end of her pregnancy:

> I just blew up like a balloon. I gained 50 pounds. And I was eating well; I was working the whole time; I worked right up until the very end [as the owner of a retail store]. I was walking and exercising. It seemed like in spite of everything, I just blew up. And then it became uncomfortable, to the point where my whole body just seemed like it didn't fit anymore. I felt like, "This isn't meant to be." I couldn't wear any of my rings or my shoes.

Even in cases like Anna's and Colleen's, edema is usually more uncomfortable than threatening. However, in some cases, it has been associated with such pregnancy-related conditions as Bell's palsy (see Chapter 7), carpal tunnel syndrome (Chapter 12), and nasal or ear congestion (Chapter 8).

However, fluid retention is most likely to make itself apparent in the feet and legs. Water, after all, flows downhill. Blood and other fluids pool in the lower extremities because forcing liquids uphill is sometimes more work than the body can handle. The collection of fluid in the feet and legs, which some authors estimate occurs in 70 percent of pregnant woman, is at least partly to blame for the changes in shoe size some women experience (see Chapter 10).

Dana said:

> I didn't realize my ankles were swelling until I was with my sister, and she said, "Look how swollen your ankles are!" And I said, "What about them?" And she said, "Look at mine." I looked at hers, and she had, like, bones sticking out! And mine didn't. But it had happened so gradually, I really didn't realize it.
>
> I made a mistake during that pregnancy. I went out and bought four pairs of shoes. And after the pregnancy was over I couldn't wear those shoes anymore because my feet had gone back to normal size.

Treatment of edema in pregnancy should be extremely conservative. The body is apparently required to gain those six to eight liters of additional fluid during pregnancy, and it is probably neither possible nor desirable to remove much of that fluid. However, in cases where fluid accumulation in tissue may be responsible for disabling conditions such as carpal tunnel syndrome, it may be worth a gentle attempt to encourage that fluid to pass back into the blood vessels, which will then carry it to the kidneys for excretion.

This movement of fluid from tissue to blood vessels to kidneys is called *diuresis*, and it may be accomplished by both chemical and mechanical means. However, chemical diuresis in pregnancy is generally not recommended. (Even in treatment of serious complications such as toxemia the effectiveness of diuretics has never been proved.) In any case, no diuretic should be taken without the guidance of a physician, including over-the-counter preparations such as Pamprin.

On the other hand, the nonpharmaceutical, mechanical treatments for edema are not only effective and without apparent risk to the baby, but downright pleasurable. First, if you can find the time, get some pillows and put your feet up. The most common prescription for dependent edema (occurring in the dependent, or hanging-down, extremities) is elevation of the feet and legs or just plain bed rest. Any supine position allows gravity to work for you instead of against you, reducing its force on the lengthy columns of veins that the blood must travel and so decreasing the pressure in the capillaries that causes water to filter into the tissues.[1] Fluid in the tissues is reabsorbed into the blood vessels, which can then transport it to the kidneys for excretion.

In the last few years, researchers at the University of North Carolina have been studying the effectiveness of another treatment for the edema of pregnancy. In one study they measured the diuretic effect of three treatments: bed rest, sitting in a bathtub with water to the waist (two to three inches below the top of the tub), and sitting in shoulder-deep water in a special immersion tank. Each treatment was undertaken for fifty minutes. In both the bathtub and the tank, the water was about 90 degrees, a temperature determined to be *thermoneutral*, feeling neither hot nor cold, for pregnant women. The results showed that diuresis was significantly greater after the shoulder-deep immersion than after either bathtub immersion or bed rest. The urine of study subjects (who emptied their bladders before each trial period) was greater not only in volume but in dilution, a key measure of how much fluid was mobilized out of the tissues into the excretory system.[2]

To be safe, a treatment for edema in pregnancy must move fluid without disturbing the electrolyte balance of the blood. A treatment that caused a significant drop in the blood levels of sodium, potassium, or other essential elements could create problems for both mother and fetus. To determine whether immersion is safe in this regard, the UNC researchers measured electrolyte levels and found that immersion produced no significant changes. These authors cite previous findings that the body adapts to the diuresis of immersion with hormonal changes that prevent the loss of electrolytes even as they allow the movement of fluid.[3]

The amount of urine the eleven women voided after immersion varied widely; the simple explanation was that women with more edema had greater diuresis. In other words, the more you pit, the more you pee. This finding, coupled with the safety and pleasure of immersion, suggests it beats all as a treatment for edema in pregnancy.

So where does the average pregnant woman find a shoulder-deep immersion tank? It's as close as the nearest swimming pool. The UNC studies state that immersion in a swimming pool produces the same diuretic effect. You don't have to be sitting still, either; the researchers recommend water aerobics, which are equally effective for diuresis. If you are already setting time aside for exercise, using that time for a water aerobics class could offer the extra benefit of relieving edema without immobilizing you in a feet–up position.

Lest you need any more convincing that water and pregnant women belong together, think about it this way: The baby inside you is floating all the time, and from his or her view, pregnancy is no doubt a pretty terrific experience. Isn't it time that you claimed for yourself at least a little of the comfort you are offering your growing child?

Now, good luck finding a bathing suit.

14

Bowel Problems

I ONCE HAD A BOYFRIEND WHOSE USUAL counsel in times of trouble was, "Don't get your bowels in an uproar." This probably goes a long way toward explaining why he never made it to husband status with me, but if he did marry, I hope he found better words of consolation before his wife bore them any children. The two most common bowel problems in pregnancy, constipation and diarrhea, are anything but uproariously funny.

Constipation

Standard obstetrical texts have two standard ideas regarding constipation: first, that most pregnant women have it; and second, that there is no need for further remarks on this "minor" complaint. Both of these assumptions are highly questionable. First, although reliable research is scanty, the few existing studies on the actual incidence of constipation in pregnancy do not show anything like an overwhelming majority of women suffering this complaint. An oft-quoted 1984 study claims 38 percent,[1] but a study from a decade before showed not only fewer cases of constipation, at 11 percent, but quite a large number of women suffering diarrhea instead.[2] Second and perhaps more important, many of the women who do experience constipation in pregnancy find it extremely upsetting and even disrupting to their daily life, suggesting that the subject merits more extensive remarks than obstetrical training tends to accord it.

One reason for the lack of accurate figures is the lack of an accurate definition of constipation. Is the definition based only on frequency of bowel movements, on their consistency, or on the difficulty of passage? And who, apart from the researchers who count these things, cares? The fact is, the feeling of constipation is highly recognizable, and you don't have to count bowel movements to know you've got it. Among the characteristics that tend to be associated with constipation—any or all of which can produce that recognizable feeling—are bloating, gas, abdominal pain, loss of appetite, and headache. It is also common to feel that the bowels have not really emptied even after a movement. The general perception of fullness and stagnation makes constipation particularly miserable for a pregnant woman, already feeling swollen and stuffy from the tip of her reddened nose (proliferation of blood vessels) to the soles of her mysteriously enlarged feet (fluid retention and fat deposits). Add the problem of getting hard bowel movements past hemorrhoids and constipation is truly no minor matter, as Kim D. noted:

> Constipation was a *big* problem with both of my pregnancies. I was drinking at least three glasses of Metamucil a day with Rachel, and it still didn't soften me up much. I switched to FiberCon with Carly. It was better but not a whole lot. I walked two miles about three times a week; I ate lettuce and anything I could think of to get me "moving." I even ate a whole can of corn one day for dinner. It worked, but not as well as I had hoped. I never really "softened." It was mostly toward the end of each pregnancy—from about six and a half months until each baby was almost six weeks old. Hemorrhoids don't help, by the way!

Like the textbook coverage, many of the theories that propose to explain constipation in pregnancy are based more on assumption than on research. However, since the path of food from the stomach to the great outdoors is not a matter of dispute, we can at least begin with some anatomical facts.

Once food leaves the stomach, it passes first through some twenty feet of coiled small intestine and then through about five feet of large intestine; what remains after this journey is solid waste. The real business of digestion, absorbing nutrients and passing them to the bloodstream, takes place in the small intestine. The main function of the large intestine is to draw water from the remaining waste before it leaves the body. As all of this is accomplished, the intestines, which are composed of smooth muscle tissue, are contracting rhythmically in an action called *peristalsis*, which moves the food along the path.

Research suggests that pregnancy may affect these digestive processes in two ways. First, the amount of water absorbed from the waste may be increased by the tendency of the entire body to retain more fluid in pregnancy. Second, it is fairly well established that the hormones of pregnancy, in protecting the uterus from untimely contractions, exert their influence over all other smooth muscle tissue, including the digestive tract. That influence may slow or disrupt the rhythm of peristalsis, causing the food to pass more slowly through the intestines. Not only would this action cause infrequent bowel movements, but it could add to the problem of excess fluid being drawn from the wastes, since the longer the material is retained in the large intestine, the more fluid will be absorbed from it.

Another organ composed of smooth muscle tissue that may be affected by progesterone is the gallbladder, which contributes to intestinal motility (ability to move) by releasing bile. Studies have established that bile flow is impaired in pregnancy. Researchers suspect that progesterone may impair the contractility of the gallbladder, resulting in an inadequate flow of bile.

The idea that progesterone is a hormonal contributor to constipation has won fairly wide acceptance in the medical literature on the strength of its apparent logic. It is not, however, established as fact. Many of the studies of the effects of progesterone on smooth muscle tissue have been conducted on rats and guinea pigs, and findings in human subjects have not always supported the assumption that what's true for rodents is true for people. Further, even if the effect were demonstrated beyond doubt, researchers might not be able to determine exactly how it happens. So far, the exact actions of progesterone on the gastrointestinal tract remain fairly mysterious.

Second in popularity to the progesterone theory but even less supported by evidence is the assumption that inadequate dietary fiber causes or contributes to constipation in pregnancy. The very small body of research on this subject has turned up only the observation by researcher Annie S. Anderson that there does not seem to be any significant difference in the fiber intake of constipated and nonconstipated pregnant women.[3] The fact that a number of subjects in Anderson's study were eating a somewhat low-fiber diet without suffering constipation suggests that lack of fiber is probably not the main reason for constipation in pregnancy.

The same study found that the fluid intakes of constipated women were significantly lower than the nonconstipated group, which suggests possible support for those who suggest extra fluids. This faction holds that a pregnant woman's fluid intake may be inadequate because the body absorbs more fluid in pregnancy and perhaps because she may be tempted to restrict fluid intake to keep from peeing all the time. Anderson's study, however, notes that so far the scientific evidence does not support the recommendation of extra fluid as a cure for pregnancy constipation.

Still other theories involve body mechanics—changes in the musculoskeletal system. For example, the uterus puts pressure on the back and abdominal muscles used for defecation; this pressure may create difficulty in pushing bowel movements out of the body. The uterus or fetal head may also put pressure on the rectum and interfere with the urge to push. Then again, perhaps the difficulty comes from weakened muscles in the pelvic floor.

Interference may also come from another quarter. If you are troubled by hemorrhoids, the pain of defecation (especially if your movements are, as Kim D. described, "a pinecone dump–ugh!") can cause your anal sphincters to develop minds of their own. Expecting pain from bowel movements does not generate enthusiasm among the appropriate muscles. Your reluctance to risk that pain may cause your lower quarters to tense and resist even when you devoutly wish a bowel movement. In cases like this, treatment of the hemorrhoids will help more than treatment of constipation, though stool softeners will ease the passage.

Feeling Better

Dietary changes. If you have been experiencing constipation, chances are that by now you have already heard the standard offering from your OB, centering largely around the addition of fiber and fluids to your diet. What your doctor may not say is how much fiber you need even to stand a chance of relief. Research has demonstrated that 27 grams of fiber per day is an effective amount for many pregnant women.[4] To give you an idea of what this means in your diet, a one-cup serving of Kellogg's Strawberry Squares (a Shredded Wheat-type cereal) contains 5 grams of dietary fiber; a slice of whole wheat bread, about 2 grams; a four-ounce serving of boiled brussel sprouts, about 4.5 grams; and a dose of a bulk supplement may contain anywhere from 2 grams (Citrucel) to 6 grams (Konsyl). Even with this much fiber, your bowel habits may not change for some time–perhaps more time than you have left in the pregnancy if your constipation has been a late-breaking story. According to one paper, the lower intestine does not fully adjust to changes in fiber intake for weeks or even months. The author notes that changes in bowel habit with the addition of fiber involve complex changes in the action of bacteria of the lower intestine and that it takes time for the bacteria to make these adjustments. To support this assertion, he cites research finding that significant changes take at least three weeks and that the effectiveness of the high-fiber diet increases over a period of months.[5]

If you haven't got that long to wait, there are a couple of other dietary factors to think about. Two substances routinely added to pregnant women's diets are dairy products and iron supplements. It is well established that both of these substances cause constipation in many people.[6] Bran cereal may be of little use if saturated with a healthy splash of cow's milk. You might experiment with removing dairy from your diet and supplementing calcium with calcium-fortified beverages such as orange juice, soy milk, or rice milk. Tums with calcium is also recommended by many obstetricians.

As for iron, it has never been established that routine supplementation with iron is necessary or even completely safe in every pregnancy. Even the World Health Organization questions the practice and recommends that iron supplements be taken only in the second half of the pregnancy, when side effects may be reduced. If you are in your first trimester or even your last, and you feel that iron may be causing your constipation, discuss with your doctor whether your blood work really demonstrates a need for the supplement. (Every pregnant woman's blood will *look* anemic because while blood increases 50 percent, red cell mass increases only 20 percent. You could ask your doctor whether your red cell count looks worse than this difference would allow for.)

Exercise. Exercise is another frequent prescription against constipation in pregnancy. One theory holds that pregnant women tend to be more sedentary and thus more susceptible to constipation. This theory makes you wonder if the theorist ever met any pregnant women, at least within the last twenty years. Pregnant women these days seem to be working full-time jobs (including taking care of other children, a job that involves not only more than forty hours a week but unlimited opportunities for exercise) and squeezing in aerobics, swimming, or walking in every available corner. However, one study of aerobic exercise in pregnancy failed to find that exercise reduced constipation,[7] a finding consistent with Kim D.'s experience. While moderate exercise is almost always recommended in pregnancy (see Appendix), failure to achieve regular bowel movements does not necessarily indicate that you are not exercising enough.

Kegel exercises may combat constipation in pregnancy.[8] Kegels, as you know if you've been attending childbirth classes, are recommended for strengthening the pelvic floor muscles in preparation for labor. They are also reported useful in relieving constipation and pelvic or rectal pain, as well as preventing bladder or bowel incontinence. Kegel exercises consist of simply tightening and releasing the muscles you would use to stop urinating. To do a Kegel, just pretend you are trying to stop a urine stream. Hold that muscle tight for ten seconds, then relax for ten seconds. Try to repeat the sequence three times. Concentrate on isolating the muscle—make sure you're not contracting muscles in your abdomen, legs, or buttocks. Do these a few times a day. They are particularly useful for passing time while waiting at red lights or sitting through television commercials.

Medications. One of the few studies of the incidence of constipation in pregnancy found that 110 of 1,000 subjects experienced a diminished bowel frequency. Although only 30 of these considered themselves constipated, 15 of those 30 mentioned that they had used laxatives.[9] In other words, at least 50 percent of the self-described constipated group felt the need for medication, suggesting that constipation in pregnancy is like the little girl with the curl in the middle of her forehead: When it's bad, it's horrid. Small wonder that you may have found yourself drawn to the laxative aisle of the drugstore—where anxiety over choosing well from a mind-boggling array of medications may have threatened to lock up your bowels for good. Unfortunately, the medical literature is not entirely consistent in its recommendations for laxatives in pregnancy. There are, however, some unanimous green and red lights, and an overview of current recommendations may provide you with a good base for discussion of the subject with your doctor.

Bulking agents. Preparations such as Metamucil and FiberCon are intended as a quick way of adding large amounts of fiber to the diet. The benefit of bulking supplements is probably not the fiber's ability to hold water—most of the fiber is broken down by the time it passes through the colon—but the fact that the fiber promotes the growth of bacteria in the colon.[10] (Bacteria are about 80 percent water, so that a stool rich in bacteria would be moist.) Nevertheless, the fiber does absorb a lot of water before reaching the colon, so when taking a bulking agent it's important to follow the directions for liquid consumption to compensate for that absorption. (Too little liquid can cause the fiber to obstruct the intestine.) Apart from this caution, the literature is apparently in agreement on the safety of bulking agents for use in pregnancy. However, remember that despite the "12 to 24 hours" notation on most of these preparations, studies mentioned above indicate that significant improvement with dietary fiber appears to take at least three weeks. Whether the time frame is shorter for concentrated bulking agents than for high-fiber foods is not clear from any remarks in the literature.

After agreeing with each other on bulking agents, doctors begin to drift apart on the subject of other laxatives. One view holds that because constipation occurs in the large intestine, medications should be limited to those with action specific to that site.[11] This caution seems particularly appropriate for pregnant women, as preparations acting in the small intestine may interfere with the absorption of nutrients. For the sake of discussion, however, here are some comments on the other readily available laxatives.

Stool softeners. These work by helping the stool hold more water . Colace (docusate sodium) and Surfak (docusate calcium) are two popular examples, and generic versions are also available. These can be purchased over the counter, but check with your doctor before taking any. The literature states that stool softeners are widely used in pregnancy without evidence of harm, but they are not well studied for safety. They may be particularly helpful if you are suffering from hemorrhoids. Be aware that some products combine stool softeners with laxatives. If you want only a softener, read packages carefully.

Lubricants. Mineral oil is probably the best known lubricant. It simply greases the skids to make the stool's passage easier. It is not absorbed by the body—but then, neither are a lot of the things you eat while you're taking it. Mineral oil is *not* recommended for use in pregnancy because it interferes with the absorption of nutrients from the small intestine, especially fat-soluble vitamins.

Osmotics. In this group fall magnesium preparations, such as Haley's M-O and Milk of Magnesia, lactulose (Chronulac), and products less common to drugstore shelves such as sorbitol and mannitol. These work by changing osmotic pressures, causing the small intestine to retain water—but it also retains nutrients that should be passing into the bloodstream, which is not desirable in pregnancy. Osmotics flunk the site-specific test because the action is in the small, not the large, intestine, and they carry a risk of serious side effects. In recent literature, only one paper recommends Milk of Magnesia in pregnancy,[12] while another notes that the risk-benefit ratio for Milk of Magnesia has not been determined and advises caution (the FDA places this drug in category C2, meaning that studies on fetal effects are not available).[13] Taken together, the writing on osmotics suggests that pregnant women would do better to avoid these laxatives.

Polyphenolic drugs. Anything with phenolphthalein (such as Ex-Lax) or bisacodyl (such as Dulcolax) is within this category. These drugs do work in the large intestine (though not all are limited to that site). They cause the colon to secrete fluids and electrolytes into its cavity. They may also affect the motor activity of the colon. Bisacodyl and phenolphthalein are both FDA category B1: Animal studies have not demonstrated a fetal risk, but the drugs have not been adequately studied in human females. Medical literature states that the risk-benefit ratio for first-trimester pregnancy has not been established but that the benefits of using the drug in the second or third trimester may outweigh the risks. This is hardly a ringing endorsement and suggests you still may wish to look elsewhere.

Senna. A naturally occurring substance, senna (Senokot) induces secretion of fluid but does not appear to affect the permeability of the large intestine (the drug is not absorbed in the small intestine). Exactly how senna works is not known, but it appears to influence motility of the large intestine. This makes the drug a great favorite with proponents of large-intestine medications, who claim that by promoting colonic motility it simply enhances the natural digestive process.[14] Nevertheless, the drug is in the same FDA category as the phenolphthaleins and carries the same risk-benefit ratio.[15] Further, holistic health advocates and herbalists frown upon the use of senna in pregnancy, reminding us that not everything that occurs naturally is intended to be taken into the body (and some substances appropriate at other times are contraindicated during pregnancy).

Other plant remedies. There appears to be universal agreement that pregnant women should not use castor oil or cascara sagrada to combat constipation. Cascara sagrada (one brand name is Nature's Remedy Natural Vegetable Laxative) is in the same class as senna (anthranoids), along with aloe, frangula, and rhubarb. A popular herbal manual[16] counsels against the use of aloe as well as flax seed and buckthorn. However, the manual does suggest that rhubarb be added to the diet. Pie, anyone?

Habit. Some doctors blame "psychosocial factors" for constipation in pregnancy. Usually, this term refers to features in the social environment that affect one's psychological functioning. It is hard to imagine how constipation in pregnancy might be produced by the social environment, unless your toilet has recently been moved to the middle of a busy public thoroughfare. That anyone should make this association only goes to show there is probably no pregnancy complaint that someone hasn't dismissed as "all in the head."

Nevertheless, though your constipation is probably not caused by psychological factors, some psychological engineering may provide a little benefit in the battle of the bowels. First of all, if you do see it as a battle, surrender. If you have tried fiber, fluids, exercise, and laxatives without success, the forces causing your constipation are apparently, like so many pregnancy symptoms, beyond your control. Admitting the temporary ascendancy of your colon will at least relieve you of the feeling that you are doing something wrong.

Second, try if at all possible to schedule a quiet, extended time (at least ten minutes, but maybe even twenty) to sit on the toilet at the same time every day. The idea is just to sit, occupying your mind with some reading material, without attempting to have a bowel movement. With luck, your body will eventually take the hint and begin responding at this time. This technique is part of the behavior modification treatment that physicians use for children who develop constipation by holding back bowel movements, and there's no reason why it shouldn't encourage movements in adults as well. Unfortunately, simple as it sounds, it is often very difficult for an adult to fit a quiet potty time into her schedule. While most people find that bowel movements are stimulated by eating in the morning, most also find that getting to work on time doesn't leave much room for contemplative bathroom study. If you have children, it is probably almost impossible for you to spend any time in the bathroom without someone pounding on the door, asking if you'll be through soon, or simply walking in and saying, "Play with me, Mommy." This is not a climate that encourages the bowels to function.

If mornings are too hectic, you might try scheduling your bathroom time after the world has gone to bed. The regularity of the hour and the freedom from disturbance are more important than the time of day. However, because the bowel is stimulated by eating and drinking, you will probably get the best results if you have a snack or a cup of hot herbal tea about 30 minutes before a nightly bathroom time.

Whether this works for your bowels or not (and remember, you're not supposed to care if it does—you're psyching your bowels out), if you succeed in incorporating these ten or twenty minutes of solitude into your daily routine, you have achieved a minor miracle, with the added benefit of some time to read the newspaper. This being the case, when delivery resolves your constipation, you may decide to keep that little secret just between you and the porcelain. With a baby in the house, twenty minutes by yourself in a tile chamber can be as great a gift as a day on the beach at Saint Thomas.

Diarrhea

The authors of a study on bowel habit in pregnancy were surprised to find that 34.4 percent of subjects experienced an increase in bowel frequency instead of the anticipated decrease (11 percent). Nearly 5 percent of subjects stated that they had experienced two to eight weeks of diarrhea toward the end of pregnancy.[17] If diarrhea is a fairly common symptom and more women actually experience bowel frequency than constipation, why do these symptoms so rarely appear in a list of pregnancy complaints?

Quite simply, the study's authors believe, because women with loose bowels don't complain. "We got the impression," they write, "that those having diarrhea regarded it as a blessing and did not consult their physician."[18] When every source from books to laxative ads leads a woman to expect constipation in pregnancy, she can feel pretty darn lucky to be running to the toilet every few hours. "To this day," wrote Kim D., who suffered severe constipation in pregnancy, "I still refuse to ever complain about being too loose, because I remember all too well how it was to be constipated."

Since diarrhea seems to be rarely reported in pregnancy, little research exists on the symptom. So far there are no studies whatsoever focusing on the incidence of diarrhea in pregnancy.[19] There are also very few attempts to explain how it occurs.

The study that revealed a frequency of diarrhea was conducted in Israel, and the authors speculate that perhaps pregnant women in that country increased their consumption of the abundantly available fruits and vegetables, leading to increased bowel frequency. However, they also note that women who significantly changed their diets were excluded from the study, meaning that none of their subjects noted a major increase in fruit and vegetable consumption.[20] Since available evidence suggests that minor changes in diet are not likely to relieve constipation, one wonders how they could possibly produce diarrhea.

Too, many women experience loose bowels in the first trimester, before diet changes might take effect, as Kate reported:

> Before I knew I was pregnant, I spent one weekend sick with really annoying diarrhea and sort of a sloshing stomach. Looking back, I think that happened about two days after conception. I don't think it was a stomach virus that just happened to occur at that time. I've never felt that way at any other time in my life.

First-trimester symptoms of pregnancy can almost always be attributed to the massive hormonal changes of that period. Early diarrhea and loose bowels are probably not exceptions. However, the Israeli study notes the possibility that diarrhea in late pregnancy may be caused by the same mechanical factor blamed for constipation, namely the gravid uterus placing pressure on the colon. While the standing assumption is that such pressure impairs bowel movements, these authors speculate that it might actually stimulate the bowels to move more frequently.

In any case but pregnancy, it might seem absurd to suggest that one factor could produce two completely opposing reactions. Perhaps it is absurd; after all, the pressure of the uterus is not a demonstrated cause of either constipation or increased bowel frequency, and one side or the other may simply be making an incorrect assumption. On the other hand, there are other factors in pregnancy—mostly hormonal—that have proved capable of producing wildly varying and even opposing reactions from woman to woman.

Diarrhea in pregnancy may often be a coincidental infection with the same agents that cause diarrhea in the general population, such as salmonella, shigella, and viruses.[21] Unfortunately, many of the medications normally prescribed for infectious diarrhea, including metronidazole, sulfa drugs, tetracycline, and quinoline drugs, carry some element of risk to the fetus. For this reason, your doctor's first response to diarrhea may be conservative treatment such as fluid replacement and Kaopectate, therapies directed at relieving the symptoms rather than toward a specific infection. If diarrhea does not respond to these measures within ninety-six hours, your doctor may want to perform a stool culture for parasitic infection. If infection exists, there are some antibiotics generally considered safe for use in pregnancy; the literature cites erythromycin and ampicillin as potentially useful and likely safe.[22]

Prolonged diarrhea that is not caused by infection could also be caused by your diet. Ingestion of cow's milk, though it causes constipation in many people, can cause loose stools, bloating, and cramping in others. Lately there has been a lot of press coverage about sensitivity to the sugar *lactose*, but probably the more common sensitivity is to the proteins in cow's milk. These proteins can pass undigested through the walls of the intestine to cause symptoms such as diarrhea. Products designed to aid digestion of dairy products by breaking down lactose, such as Lact-Aid milk, will not provide any relief to persons sensitive to cow's milk proteins. If you have been flooding your system with dairy products in order to keep up your calcium intake, you might consider dropping all dairy from your diet for a week or two. Supplement with other calcium sources (calcium-fortified orange juice, soy milk, rice milk, or Tums with calcium) in the meantime, and wait to see if the diarrhea improves. If it does, you have the opportunity for further experimenting. Try dairy again. Does the diarrhea return? Go back to your substitute calcium sources.

Finally, diarrhea close to term may be an indication that labor is approaching. The reigning assumption regarding bowel habit during pregnancy is that gastrointestinal action is slowed by hormonal effects. Sudden diarrhea in the last trimester may suggest a hormonal change preceding labor.[23] While the researchers emphasize that diarrhea in pregnancy is not usually a sign of preterm labor, it certainly can't hurt to check with your doctor if you experience a sudden attack near term.

As noted above, standard and conservative treatment for diarrhea in pregnancy usually involves fluid replacement; possibly, the addition of lactobacillus to the diet; and the use of antidiarrheals such as kaolin or pectin (Kaopectate), which reduce bowel movement frequency by absorbing water in the large intestine. Because these medications are not absorbed by the body, they are believed to be safe in pregnancy. Medications to avoid include anything that is absorbed by the digestive system, including diphenoxylate with atropine (Lomotil), which has been associated with malformations in human infants with first-trimester use; bismuth subsalicylate (Pepto-Bismol), because salicylates (aspirin) have caused birth defects in animals and hemorrhages in newborn babies; and loperamide (Imodium), the safety of which has not been established in pregnancy.

The good news about diarrhea and constipation in pregnancy is that both will resolve after delivery. The bad news is that after delivery you may have whole days when you cannot find a moment to use the bathroom. Like constipation and diarrhea, this is a minor problem only in the eyes of those with no experience in the matter. But unlike these, it can be cleared up with a little education of the parties involved.

15

Skin Problems

YOU CAN PUT UP WITH A LITTLE BLOSSOMING acne. You can maturely accept as a common feature of pregnancy the fact that your skin has darkened over your cheeks and nose, even though every time you look in the mirror you want to yell, "Hi, ho, Silver." You have even made your peace with stretch marks. However your outermost layer happens to reflect your gravid state, you could learn to live with it . . . if you could *just stop this itching*.

Christy related this helpful exchange with her OB:

> I had a rash on the tops of my thighs, and it itched a whole lot. I asked my doctor, "Is this due to changes in hormone levels?" And he said, "I don't know. I don't do rashes." He just saw it as not pregnancy related, and it wasn't an issue we were going to cover that day. . . . So I just tried to ignore it. I didn't do anything.

Despite the convictions of Christy's doctor, the medical literature lists no fewer than six specific dermatoses (skin disorders) unique to pregnancy, and three of these itch so much that *pruritic*—docspeak for "itchy"—is the first word in their names. Descriptions of the others usually mention itching as the primary symptom. Also, preexisting skin disorders that produce itching can be exacerbated by pregnancy. And systemic problems, most commonly liver dysfunction associated with pregnancy, can produce intense itching in the absence of any rash. One study estimates that itching occurs in 3 to 14 percent of pregnancies,[1] but conversations with groups of pregnant women suggest this is an underestimate. Most likely, if you once thought you had an itch to bear a child, you didn't know the half of it until now.

Pregnancy produces significant changes in the skin, well beyond the expected (and still largely unexplained) stretch marks. Skin changes begin very early with the increase in blood volume, which causes distention in blood vessels throughout the body. Further distention occurs when the growing uterus, compressing the inferior vena cava (which receives blood from the lower half of the body), begins to impair the return of blood to the heart. Normal pregnancy is a low blood pressure state, and by the second half the blood vessels have simply lost much of the squeezing power that normally forces the blood along its proper course. Meanwhile, pregnancy is also a proliferative state in which rapid cell reproduction causes significant growth of new tissue, and to supply that tissue your body is rapidly spinning new webs of tiny vessels just under the skin surface. Consequently, blood flow in the skin is significantly increased—the origin, no doubt, of that hideous cliché about glowing.

The increased volume of blood, moving relatively slowly through an unusual number of fragile new blood vessels, is bringing excessive amounts of hormones to skin cells that are likely already primed to react to those hormones. According to recent studies the skin cells of pregnant women and users of oral contraceptives have more than the normal amount of receptors for estrogens and progesterone.[2] Receptors are sites where molecules can latch onto cell membranes like keys fitting into locks. When the molecules bind themselves to cells in this way, various reactions are permitted. This increase in skin cell receptors for steroids is otherwise most commonly seen in patients with skin cancer (another state of excess proliferation).

Altogether, the new tissue growth, new blood vessels, increased blood volume with slower flow, and cell priming leave the skin a well-prepared canvas on which the little dramas of pregnancy—immune reactions, hormonal sensitivities, systemic dysfunctions—may be painted in the most florid colors. Some or all of these conditions may also predispose to itching.

Hormones have a demonstrated effect on certain disorders of the skin. It was noted as early as 1929 that subjects with an itching dermatitis known as *Besnier's prurigo* experienced more severe symptoms prior to menstruation. Similarly, both menstruation and pregnancy have been linked to flare-ups of the itchy, scaly skin disorder known as *atopic dermatitis.*[3]

Even without a rash, hormones may simply make you itch more. Research demonstrates that the *itch/pain threshold*—the amount of stimulation required for the body to note and respond to the signals of itch or pain—varies according to the phases of the menstrual cycle (the greatest sensitivity occurring between ovulation and the menstrual period). Further research suggests that premenstrual exacerbation of itching, along with other cyclical variations such as increased redness and rash produced by contact with certain allergens, may indicate an autoimmune response in which the body reacts to its own production of progesterone.[4]

This research seems relevant to the experience of Linda M., who reported that her pregnancy provoked an allergic reaction to substances that had never bothered her before:

> I developed a severe allergy to detergent and ended up at the dermatologist having biopsies to rule out autoimmune disorders. This happened in the middle trimester. I feel if I hadn't been at a major medical center, they would have said, "It's a rash. Change detergents." But at UNC, they've seen *everything*, and so they knew what horrible things it could be. It was scary, but I realized this pregnancy was worth lupus or whatever. When they determined it was nothing, I felt I would gladly scratch in peace. Then it went away. It probably took a little while to get all the detergent residue from my clothes, and I think I reacted to the hydrocortisone cream as well.

Certainly the demonstrated influence of hormones on allergic reactions could have been a factor in Linda's case.

Besides bringing hormones in contact with skin cells, the increased blood volume and slowed flow of pregnancy likely predispose to itching in other ways. First of all, pressure from distended blood vessels can stimulate nerve endings. Sometimes this stimulation may produce pain, a mechanism proposed as the cause of pregnancy-related night backache (see Chapter 5). In the skin, which is rich with nerve endings that can transmit a variety of sensations depending on the pattern of stimulation, pressure from blood vessels may telegraph itch to the brain. Further, because blood flow is sluggish, metabolic products that would otherwise be cleared from the blood may instead accumulate and irritate nerve fibers.

Increased blood volume and slower flow are *physiologic* responses to pregnancy—that is, the body is functioning in a manner that is normal under a given circumstance. Sometimes, however, the body's attempts to adapt to pregnancy produce an exaggerated reaction, such as a skin rash. While such reactions are common, it is worth remembering that *common* is not the same thing as *normal*. Actual dermatoses, whether well recognized or highly individual, represent at least some degree of disorder. For this reason they merit full attention for what they reveal about how the human body struggles to adapt to pregnancy. They also deserve thorough and sympathetic consideration by your health practitioner, since (depending on their severity) they may significantly disrupt your health or routine.

Pruritic Urticarial Papules and Plaques of Pregnancy (PUPPP)

Translated, the descriptive name of this disorder means "itchy, hivelike, raised bumps and patches seen only in pregnant women." The rash usually appears late in the third trimester—the average is thirty-six weeks—and most commonly (in 76 percent of cases, according to a study by the National Institutes of Health) in first pregnancies. The lesions usually begin on the abdomen as little pimplelike bumps, and as if to add insult to injury, they tend at first to localize along and around any stretch marks. As the rash progresses, it often forms clusters—a diagnostic sign for a doctor trying to distinguish it from other rashes. It may also move across the abdomen and chest, the arms and legs, and the buttocks, but almost never does it appear above the breasts or on the face. Sometimes the lesions are filled with fluid, making them resemble tiny blisters.

Above all, whatever it may look like, this rash itches severely. Many women complain of sleep disturbance or disruption of daily routines.

Though medical papers unvaryingly refer to PUPPP as the most common dermatosis of pregnancy, this disorder and its description appeared in the literature only in 1979,[5] which makes one wonder whether doctors before that time were paying attention. A more generous speculation is that they were misdiagnosing it as something previously recognized (such as *herpes gestationis*, discussed later in this chapter) or calling it by a different name.[6] (Various authors list *toxemic rash of pregnancy, papular dermatitis of pregnancy, Bourne's toxemic rash, toxic erythema of pregnancy,* and *Nurse's late prurigo of pregnancy* as possibly identical to PUPPP.) Even now, the medical community is not entirely sold on the PUPPP label. Some writers refer instead to *polymorphic eruption of pregnancy* (*polymorphic* meaning "having many forms"), a name suggested in 1983.[7]

Despite the arguments it provoked, the naming of this dermatosis in 1979 at least inspired recognition of the disorder as a clinical entity, opening the way to research into its causes. So far, that research has resulted in about as much clarity and agreement as the search for a name. Some theories have died on the vine when studies failed to support hypotheses; others have been plucked and stomped upon by researchers who failed to reproduce others' findings or who simply find the theories illogical.

Because it appears only in pregnancy, researchers have examined possible roles for various hormones in causing the disorder. No study thus far has revealed any association between unusual hormone levels and PUPPP. Studies have also examined PUPPP as a possible autoimmune disorder—that is, an allergic reaction to a substance produced by the mother's body. Again, no study has posted any promising results; most find no evidence of any immune reaction.

Focusing on the common elements of PUPPP–its association with first pregnancy, the tendency of the lesions to localize on stretch marks, and the reported increased incidence with twin pregnancies, large weight gain, and large newborn weight–one group of researchers developed a theory that rapid abdominal stretching creates some sort of trauma to the skin, triggering an inflammatory response that appears as the lesions of PUPPP.[8] Detractors, however, point out that other conditions may cause rapid stretching of the abdomen without producing anything like PUPPP. Perhaps the stretch marks only offer the lesions an easy location for eruption.

A much more exotic and interesting theory has recently issued forth from a pair of South African doctors who had the good fortune to observe PUPPP in patients with unusual familial relationships that offered some intriguing possibilities. In each case, a pair of sisters married a pair of brothers. (In one case, both the wives and the husbands were identical twins.) In each case, both sisters developed PUPPP. The doctors believe that these cases combined suggest a genetic factor in PUPPP–specifically, that the father, in fertilizing the egg, may contribute a substance that produces an allergic reaction in the mother. Perhaps, they suggest, this substance does not exert its influence until late in pregnancy, or perhaps it is not released into the mother's circulation until the placenta begins to degenerate toward delivery (which would explain the characteristically late occurrence of the rash). This theory holds up better than a possible alternative, namely that the mothers in these cases shared a genetic predisposition to develop PUPPP. There are few other reported cases of PUPPP occurring among related females.[9]

Whatever the controversy surrounding PUPPP, researchers are in agreement over its course: quick resolution following delivery. The rash or redness may be visible for two or three weeks after the birth, but the itching tends to disappear more quickly. Because the rash tends to start so late in pregnancy and resolve thereafter, its course is altogether fairly quick–which is all to the good, as finding relief can be difficult. A report on twenty-five subjects noted that a number of remedies had been tried without success: antihistamines, barbiturates, vitamin E creams, cocoa butter, calamine lotion, and moisturizing lotions. However, most of the subjects did obtain some relief from skin creams containing hydrocortisone.[10] You can discuss these topical corticosteroid creams with your physician, but don't use them on your own, even though many are available over the counter.

Herpes Gestationis

After PUPPP, the dermatosis appearing most frequently in the medical literature is an itchy eruption with the frightening and inappropriate name of *herpes gestationis.* This rash is not in any way related to the herpes virus and in fact shows no evidence of viral origin. The term *herpes gestationis* was coined in the nineteenth century, when medical writers still clung to a second-century usage for the word *herpes*—from the Greek for "to creep"—to connote skin disorders, with their sometimes creeping character. Despite the different application of "herpes" today, a tradition of eighteen hundred years is apparently hard for the medical profession to shake.

There is no consensus whatever on the occurence of herpes gestationis. Estimates vary from one case in three thousand pregnancies to one in fifty thousand. The latter estimate comes from a doctor who claims that even in large urban practices, few dermatologists have ever seen the rash.[11] He does not mention how many OBs might have seen it without referring patients to dermatologists, but given the severity of this disorder—many of whose sufferers consider surgical sterilization when they learn that the disease recurs in subsequent pregnancies—it seems unlikely that any doctor would shrug this one off with the remark that he doesn't do rashes.

Extreme itching is often the first symptom of herpes gestationis, which in first pregnancies usually appears in the second or third trimester (earlier in subsequent pregnancies). The lesions tend to appear first around the navel, but the arms and legs may also be involved. Lesions may first resemble hives, but after a few days they develop into blisters. They crust over and then heal; the skin may be darkened afterward but will probably not scar.

In some patients, the skin begins to clear of these lesions as delivery approaches. However, in nearly all cases, symptoms flare again with delivery. Postpartum, the disorder resolves rather slowly. A potentially valuable piece of information for sufferers of herpes gestationis is a finding that related shorter healing time to breastfeeding. In this study, lesions cleared in an average of five to twenty-four weeks in women who breastfed their infants, while women who exclusively bottlefed continued to suffer symptoms for up to an average of sixty-eight weeks.[12]

Even after symptoms clear, the disease may flare mildly with menstruation or ovulation. Some women experience recurrences with the use of oral contraceptives. Clearly the disease favors a certain hormonal environment, but immunological testing suggests that herpes gestationis is an immune reaction to a substance as yet unknown.

A woman who suffers herpes gestationis is likely vulnerable to the offending substance (the antigen) through her genetic makeup. Further, the genes of the baby's father may increase the likelihood of a reaction. This disorder is also seen in women with *choriocarcinoma* or *hydatiform mole,* two conditions involving a fertilized egg that does not develop into a fetus. Thus the father's sperm is likely involved. As may be the case in PUPPP (discussed earlier in this chapter), perhaps the paternal contribution includes a substance to which the woman's immune system reacts at some point in the pregnancy.

Herpes gestationis is nearly always treated with oral steroids, commonly prednisone. Steroid creams are not likely to be of much help while the disease it at its peak, though they may be worth a try during menstrual recurrences, which are typically fairly mild.

A study from 1961 claims success in treating herpes gestationis with vitamin B_6.[13] This report has not been followed up in the literature of the intervening years.

Other Skin Disorders

Once you get past herpes gestationis, the medical literature becomes a bit blurry on pregnancy-associated dermatoses. The remaining distinct entity, a rare disorder called *impetigo herpetiformis* (that deceptive "herpes" label again), is not unique to pregnancy, though pregnancy seems to bring on a particularly acute phase. Beyond that there tends to be a good deal of overlap among terms and descriptions and little agreement about where one disorder ends and another begins. One wonders whether the better recognized (and supposedly rare) dermatoses might simply be exaggerated cases of many of the mild skin symptoms more commonly experienced, such as Linda B. described in her second pregnancy:

> The rash basically covered my belly. I had just started using lotions and whatnot, and I don't know what happened first—I was starting to itch a little, and I thought, "My skin's getting dry. It's time to start putting something on it." I don't know if what was making me itch was the rash that was coming on, or the rash was a reaction to a lotion. But I also put the lotion on my hands and arms, and the only place that broke out was my belly. It was red, and it wasn't quite big enough to be blisters, but they were like little tiny miniblisters. My belly wasn't completely covered, but there were a few spots here, a few spots there . . . lower than my belly button, but I also had a fair lot of it up across the top of my belly. It itched quite a bit! It started as my belly was starting to stretch a fair amount, so probably about the fifth month. I really didn't have it long, maybe a week and a half. I stopped using the lotions, but it didn't go away right after that.

Nevertheless, the dermatoses can often be divided into recognizable groups, and there is value in making the effort to distinguish among them. Some carry constitutional symptoms, so that (for example) flulike illness may actually be connected with a rash. And although no paper suggests that any of these problems poses a significant risk to the fetus, certainly anything even remotely associated with potential problems requires prompt and correct diagnosis so that treatment options can be discussed. A medication proved effective for one dermatosis may do nothing for another.

However, there is also value in considering the overall picture of skin disorders in pregnancy. Sustained study of the medical literature on the subject–after which the words themselves seem to start swelling up and bursting from the page–gives the impression that the skin of pregnant women is like a minefield, with the potential for explosions lying just beneath the surface.

The value of this perspective is the awareness it provides that the pregnant body is in a state of high stress. This awareness is definitely at odds with the romantic view of pregnancy as the female body's optimal state of functioning. If you are suffering from miserable pregnancy symptoms such as skin disorders, trying to live up to that view can place a heavy burden on your already loaded shoulders. Sometimes a realistic consideration of the stresses of pregnancy can go a long way toward lifting that burden.

Eruptions of the skin tell us that the body is struggling to accommodate an internal disruption–an upset of the usual balance, or the presence of foreign substances. Pregnancy involves both of these disruptive elements. Certainly things are out of balance, especially the hormone levels–which themselves are struggling to adapt to pregnancy, a struggle that does not always produce the levels considered normal for gestation. In keeping with this, many of the skin disorders are associated either with hormone levels considered unusual for pregnancy or with recurrences during the hormonal fluctuations of the menstrual cycle. As for foreign substances, pregnancy begins with a package of someone else's genetic material taking up residence in the mother's body. The consequences of this beginning are played out over thirty-eight to forty weeks–usually with success, but not always without incident. A lot depends on the particular combination of the mother's and father's genes. It is already well established that certain combinations can produce destructive immune responses, as is the case with Rh disease (in which the mother's body produces antibodies to a protein that the fetus inherits from the father's blood type). Perhaps significantly, a number of patients in a study of papular dermatitis of pregnancy (considered a rare disorder) were Rh-negative.[14] The fact that in such cases the father's genetic material could provoke a widely recognized reaction in the mother's immune system makes one wonder if a paternal factor could have also contributed to the skin symptoms, as has been suggested in cases of PUPPP and herpes gestationis (discussed earlier in this chapter).

The genetic component is no doubt what keeps dermatologists guessing about many pregnant women's skin symptoms. Exactly how the skin reacts depends on not just the mother's genetic makeup but the father's as well. When you consider the infinite number of possible combinations, it seems unreasonable to expect that every pregnant woman's dermatosis will fall neatly into one of six or a dozen categories.

Confusing the picture even further, the stresses of pregnancy are not limited to the immune system, and other factors can influence individual reactions to pregnancy and their manifestations on the skin. The most common example is liver dysfunction, which is due to the liver's inability to adapt to the stresses of pregnancy and which can cause severe itching without the appearance of rash or eruptions. This itching usually appears in the third trimester and may be followed by jaundice. Accompanying fatigue, nausea, vomiting, and loss of appetite have been reported, but since these symptoms are characteristic of pregnancy at any time (not just in the first trimester, as many women can attest), it is difficult to say with certainty that they are associated with the itching.

The liver dysfunction that leads to itching is called *cholestasis*, a condition caused by stagnation of bile in the liver (see Chapter 1). Women with cholestasis of pregnancy characteristically show elevated blood levels of bile salts (one of the main components of bile, helping the breakdown and absorption of fats). The presence of these salts in the skin relates proportionately to the severity of itching, suggesting that this presence is either the cause of or an influencing factor in the occurrence of pruritus. However, another possibility exists: The plasma of women with itching due to cholestasis of pregnancy has been found to contain unusually high levels of steroid metabolites. These substances are the products of the metabolism of hormones, such as the estrogens, and they in turn may be partially metabolized by the skin itself. Perhaps this metabolic action or its by-products play some role in the onset of pruritus.

Some doctors suggest that oral antihistamines or topical creams may be helpful in controlling pruritus due to cholestasis[15]; however, other authors claim a poor success rate for these medications.[16] (In any case, you should not use either without first discussing it with your doctor.) There is apparent agreement on the use, in severe cases, of a drug called *cholestyramine*. If your physician prescribes this drug (brand name Questran), ask about supplementing fat-soluble vitamins—particularly vitamin K—which are bound (made unavailable for absorption) by the drug.

Just as the absence of a rash does not preclude itching in pregnancy, the absence of itching is no guarantee that your skin will not undergo visible changes. In fact, some of the more common changes are highly visible, including edema (see Chapter 13), varicose veins (see Chapter 10), growths, and color changes (hyperpigmentation). Hair and nails usually do not escape this sometimes unwelcome makeover. Last but hardly least, there are stretch marks, probably the most common pregnancy symptom visited upon the skin.

Growths

It is not unusual to develop skin tags associated with pregnancy (*molluscum fibrosum gravidarum*). Skin tags are protruding nodes of flesh, usually from pinhead- to pea-sized, which may be either the same color as the surrounding skin or darker. They usually occur in the second half of pregnancy, turning up on the neck, in the armpits, between the breasts, and sometimes on the feet. Sometimes they regress after delivery; sometimes they hang on and get larger in subsequent pregnancies. No one knows why they form, but they are not dangerous.

Another growth that may develop during pregnancy is the *dermatofibroma*, a round or oval, reddish brown nodule. It tends to appear on the arms above the elbows or on the sides of the body. Again, this is not a sign of any dangerous skin condition.

Hyperpigmentation and Melasma

Doctors sometimes complain that it is difficult to learn much about the dermatoses of pregnancy because they rarely encounter cases for study. Yet common conditions such as hyperpigmentation—occurring in up to 90 percent of pregnant women—are often no better understood than the rare disorders despite the amount of subjects available for research. This suggests something less than alacrity and enthusiasm in the study of benign conditions. However, the dramatic changes in appearance can be unsettling—and Lisa's experience suggests that doctors should at least be well versed in the subject.

Eight to ten weeks into her first pregnancy, Lisa noticed a darkening "across the bridge of my nose and up my cheeks." Because Lisa was at the same time experiencing bouts of "strange migratory joint pain," her family physician became concerned that she might have the autoimmune disorder lupus, often characterized by a "butterfly rash" over the nose and cheeks. Lisa spent a number of days in something close to terror (days during which her doctor apparently misplaced her test results) before learning that she did not have the disease. At this point she switched to an OB-GYN for prenatal care. When she asked him about the facial coloring, he "kinda chuckled and told me it was the mask of pregnancy," she said.

Hyperpigmentation is a darkening of certain areas of the skin. In pregnancy, this darkening tends to focus on sites that are already more deeply colored than the surrounding skin, such as the areole (area around the nipples), genitals, and perineum (area between the genitals and the anus). These areas contain greater deposits of the skin-coloring pigment *melanin* than are found in the skin around them. A line running approximately from the pubic bone to the navel may also appear or, if already present, grow darker. Any other area with more than the usual amount of pigment is likewise subject to this darkening, including scars and freckles. Hyperpigmentation usually fades rapidly after delivery, but the skin in affected areas tends to remain just a bit darker than its prepregnancy color.

Researchers have not established exactly why this hyperpigmentation occurs. Naturally they suspect that hormones are responsible, but although estrogens, progesterone, and a substance called *MSH* (melanocyte-stimulating hormone) have been implicated, it is so far only an implication and not a conviction.

Melanocytes are cells that produce melanin, so something that stimulates melanocytes certainly sounds like a logical culprit. The role of MSH is particularly in dispute because it does not reach high levels until late pregnancy, whereas the hyperpigmentation begins quite early, usually in the first trimester.

Estrogens and progesterone, on the other hand, have a demonstrated relationship with *nevi*, areas of skin where new melanocytes are produced. According to recent research, pregnancy or the use of oral contraceptives tends to increase the number of estrogen and progesterone receptors on nevi cells. In other words, these cells have an increased affinity for binding with these hormones, and that binding may activate the nevi in some way to cause the hyperpigmentation. This phenomenon bears some similarity to the development of melanoma, another circumstance that increases the receptor sites for estrogens and progesterone. However, research has never established a convincing connection between pregnancy and an increased risk of developing melanoma. If you are at risk for melanoma (due to family history) you should watch your moles for surface area growth or other visible changes during your pregnancy. If you are uncertain about what to look for, consult a dermatologist. And wear sunscreen.

When hyperpigmentation occurs over the face, as in Lisa's case, it is called *melasma*, *chloasma*, or "the mask of pregnancy." This condition may occur in up to 70 percent of pregnant women of all races. It is caused by the deposit of excess melanin in either the epidermis (thin, outer cellular layer of the skin) or the dermis (inner layer, containing nerves, blood vessels, fat, and collagen and elastic fibers). Deposits in the epidermis are more common (72 percent of cases) and tend to be more noticeable, appearing light brown in natural light. The less dramatic dermal deposits appear blue-gray. (A few women also get a mixed type, with deposits in both dermis and epidermis; this type produces deep brown patches.) These melanin deposits may involve the cheeks, forehead, upper lip, nose and chin. Most cases resolve after delivery, though some color may persist for up to a year.

As in other cases of hyperpigmentation, the hormonal levels of pregnancy are thought to be responsible for melasma, but medical literature additionally stresses that the condition may be exacerbated by sun exposure. Cosmetics have been cited as a possible contributing factor (along with nutrition, liver disease, parasitic infections, and the genetic makeup of the individual).[17] If you develop melasma, by all means protect your skin with sunscreens and hats, and consider abandoning cosmetics or at least experimenting to see if a particular product seems to irritate or exacerbate the pigmented areas. You should also avoid rubbing or irritating these areas. These precautions may speed the regression of the pigment after your baby is born. You may also wish to consider that melasma sometimes persists or recurs in women who use oral contraceptives following delivery, a fact that may at least temporarily affect your choice of birth control.

If, after delivery, you are swaddling yourself like a mummy on the beach and are not using oral contraceptives yet melasma persists, some therapies are available and may be helpful. Ask your doctor (who may refer you to a dermatologist) about the following medications, each of which has been cited in the literature as having possible benefit (but remember they are appropriate only after delivery, and possibly not while breastfeeding):

hydroquinone (2–4%) cream

retinoic acid (.5%) cream

corticosteroid cream

combination: tretinoin (.1%), hydroquinone (5%), and dexamethasone (.1%) cream

Among the possible side effects of this last formulation are dermatitis (rashes), hyperpigmentation, and hypopigmentation (that is, the skin areas become paler than surrounding skin).[18]

Stretch Marks

The medical literature refers to these as either *striae distensae* (literally, "stretch marks") or *striae gravidarum* ("marks of pregnancy"). Because these marks are associated with other conditions besides pregnancy, the first term is really more accurate. However, it is the stretch marks of pregnancy that get the most attention—from everyone but most medical professionals. While a standard OB text refers to them as "trivial," stretch marks receive tremendous coverage in pregnancy books and women's magazines. (A study on a possible treatment for stretch marks was featured in the *National Enquirer* several months before it appeared in the medical literature.)[19] Evidently, stretch marks are an interesting subject to a lot of people—presumably a lot of female people with extremely distended abdomens.

Stretch marks occur in up to 90 percent of pregnant white women, less commonly among black and Asian women. They usually begin in the late second trimester as pink or violet lines in the skin of the abdomen, breasts, or thighs. They may also appear in the upper arms, lower back, buttocks, thighs, or groin. After delivery they usually fade to a lighter color, but the change to the skin is permanent—though, so far, no one knows exactly what that change is.

Among the other conditions tending to produce stretch marks are infections, rapid weight gain, and steroid-overload conditions such as Cushing's syndrome. Each of these conditions shares some feature with pregnancy—stressed immune system, rapid stretching of the skin, unusual levels of steroids—and reasonable arguments can be made for each of these features as the cause of stretch marks, especially since both hormones and stretching have demonstrated effects on the framework of connective tissue that comprises the underlying layer of the skin. However, at this point none of the scant existing research has produced any conclusions, and all medical literature still lists the cause as "obscure" or unknown.

A 1959 study associated stretch marks with glucose intolerance, based on the finding that women with stretch marks displayed lower glucose tolerance than women without.[20] This finding appeared to support the theory that stretch marks were caused by pregnancy-associated hyperactivity of the adrenal cortex, since this gland produces corticosteroids, which are among the regulators of glucose levels in the blood. (Excessive levels of corticosteroids from an overactive adrenal cortex can impair glucose tolerance.) Another study appearing to support this theory demonstrated that obese, nonpregnant women with stretch marks had higher levels of corticosteroids than those without stretch marks. However, the one study that has attempted to replicate the association between glucose intolerance and stretch marks failed to do so. The study author notes that her small sample size (forty-eight subjects) may have skewed her findings and still finds the role of adrenal cortical hyperactivity "intriguing and plausible."[21]

Perhaps the most significant finding of this study was the amount of concern women expressed over stretch marks—clear evidence that despite the pronouncements of obstetrical texts, stretch marks were not a trivial problem for those experiencing them. Sixty-three percent of subjects had attempted to prevent the formation of the marks, by application of lotions or creams or by exercising. Their concern is in keeping with the amount of attention stretch marks receive in the popular media. Magazines, pregnancy books, and television advertisements all offer advice or products intended to prevent or erase stretch marks.

Regardless of the media attention, not one of the various prescriptions has ever been proved effective in preventing stretch marks. This poor success rate is not surprising, considering that not one purported remedy is based on any knowledge of what causes stretch marks to form in the first place. Reports of success with such regimens as olive oil or cocoa butter massage, increased protein intake, or increased vitamin C or E are purely anecdotal—that is, women here and there have claimed success, but no study has demonstrated conclusive effects. After all, these methods are only supposed to be successful at *preventing* stretch marks, so who can say if they worked? If a woman uses method A or B from the early weeks of pregnancy and does not get stretch marks, perhaps she simply wouldn't have gotten them anyway.

The only treatment that has shown any promise in erasing stretch marks once they have formed is topical applications of retinoids, substances exhibiting a vitamin A-like activity. These are not to be used during pregnancy or breastfeeding as they may have serious harmful effects, so if you're bound to try them, discuss them with your doctor after delivery and weaning.

Hair and Nail Changes

"When I was about one month pregnant," said Kate, "people started noticing my hair all of a sudden, telling me it looked beautiful. I hadn't told anyone I was pregnant." She went on:

> I couldn't believe they were noticing my hair instead of the purple scars around my eyes from all the vomiting I was doing, but it's true, I did have great hair for my whole pregnancy. Then if you look at pictures of me about five months after my baby was born, I'm just about bald. I cut my hair because it looked so bad in those pictures—I thought I just had an ugly hairstyle. I didn't know that my hair was falling out and would eventually grow back normally again.

Most women experience bountiful growth of scalp hair in pregnancy. This growth has been traced to a change in the growth phases of scalp hair follicles caused by pregnancy hormones. Throughout life, each follicle on the scalp moves through phases of growth (*anangen phase*), lasting several years, and rest (*telogen phase*), lasting a few months. The follicles act independently so that most of the time you have some hairs growing and others falling out. However, in some pregnancies, more than 90 percent of scalp hair follicles suddenly shift to the anangen phase, so that hair growth is much thicker than normal. After delivery, most of those follicles shift to the telogen phase, which ends with the hair falling out. The resulting rapid hair loss, called *telogen effluvium*, usually begins one to five months after delivery and lasts up to about fifteen months.

Strangely, the hair follicles elsewhere on the body do not seem to go through the same synchronized anangen phase, yet some women experience pronounced growth of hair on the body in pregnancy. This growth may produce a sudden excess or darkening of the hair on your face, arms, legs, back, and the area above the pubic region. (Now you feel not only huge but huge and hairy. It is difficult to glow under these circumstances.) Naturally, researchers speculate that this growth is also influenced by hormones, though an unusual candidate, androgen, is sometimes nominated. Certain ovarian abnormalities associated with pregnancy may produce androgen and thus stimulate body hair growth.[22]

Androgen may also be responsible for the tendency in some women to lose hair in pregnancy, in a pattern that resembles the classic balding of men: receeding hairline at the forehead and temples as well as scattered thinning over the scalp. Whatever the cause, this hair loss usually reverts to normal after delivery, so that while every other new mother's hair is falling out, yours will be growing back in.

Changes in the nails are also common and begin early, perhaps by the sixth week. Your nails may grow more quickly than usual and may become brittle or soft. Some women see grooves developing across the nail, and the nail may even begin to separate from the finger. These changes have never been adequately explained. Expect resolution six months to a year after delivery. In the meantime, wear gloves for dishwashing, gardening, and anything else that exposes your nails to chemicals, injury, or prolonged soaking. Keep nails short and avoid nail polish. If you are taken in by suggestions to pamper yourself with some sort of beauty treatment during pregnancy, don't choose a manicure, as the changes in the nails may make the nail beds more prone to infection.

Clearly, even if your OB doesn't "do" skin problems, pregnancy *does*—with a repertoire that could shame the most versatile performer. And of course, whatever pregnancy does, you are also required to do. Do it, then, in whatever way works for you. Ignore, curse, treat—your repertoire can vary, too. With luck, you and your skin will soon be performing in harmony again.

Epilogue

"OVERALL," WROTE LINDA SUE IN HER seventh month, "my thought is, 'Why do women do this multiple times? Thus far it just doesn't feel worth it.'"

Linda Sue suffered the whole array of miserable pregnancy symptoms, including abdominal pain, backache, nausea, heartburn, edema, ear problems, fatigue, and more. "I have been told it is not terminal," she wrote, "but that is *little* comfort when you're going through it."

Why does so much of the advice you get in pregnancy seem to provide so little comfort? Undoubtedly because most of it requires perspective, and while a pregnant woman may develop keenness of other senses like taste and smell, her sense of perspective is down for the count. Betty H. told this story:

> I had the flu in my first pregnancy. Joe missed me one night in bed and got up, and I was sitting in the living room crying. And he says, "What is wrong?" And I said, "I feel terrible and I can't sleep and I've used my *last Sucret*!" To me that was the total end of the world—*I had no more Sucrets.* Everything was out of proportion.

Most pregnant women reach a point—usually around seven months—where they begin to believe they will be pregnant forever. "I was so miserable," wrote Betty W., who suffered intense nausea and vomiting. "It was hard to believe anyone who said that it would end and I'd feel human again." While most events in adult life seem to charge across the calendar like a thundering herd, being pregnant is like being stuck on the slowpoke mount that stops to crop the grass while the rest of the world races by. You become convinced that you will never see the end of this trip—and you don't even know what will be waiting for you if you do.

About the best that you can hope for to get you through pregnancy is that a few understanding types will dismount from their fast horses, walk back to you, and offer a few encouraging words to help you pass the time. No one can make that horse move any faster, but maybe the right advice will offer some real help along the way.

Sometimes, the best advice is simply to believe in yourself. Louise wrote:

> Don't assume anything is your fault, unless evidence points to that, and if it does, change your behavior. Think well of yourself, have confidence, trust in yourself, and put yourself first.

Jan echoed this advice: "Trust that there is nothing you could have done to cause the sickness or to get over it more quickly. It is not a psychological problem or a sign of weakness."

B.J., too, stressed the need to believe in and care for yourself: "Always do what you feel is right for you. Pray a lot; meditate to calming music. Get a massage. Take care of yourself, and you will be taking care of your baby."

However, you do not have to be entirely self-reliant. Seek support without hesitation or embarrassment. As Shannon wrote, "People do honestly want to help you, and you should let them." Sarah said, "Take advantage of any help, visitation, or assistance that's offered from friends or family. Cry as often as you need to. And try to communicate as openly as possible." Be especially open with your partner, as his understanding and sympathy will make the greatest difference in how you get through the difficulties day by day.

One thing that makes it so difficult to get sympathy and good advice in pregnancy is the rapid Loss of Pregnancy Memory that many women experience after delivery. Said Welmoed, "I hated hearing all these women around me gushing about how their pregnancies were like holidays. B.S.!" Linda Sue remarked that "the things of no use or that made me feel worse were comments like, 'Poor thing. I never experienced that,' or, 'Pregnancy was the best time of my life.' They must be in denial or lying through their teeth!" Probably they are simply forgetting—and with that forgetting comes the magical return of perspective. During her interview, Christy, mother of a two-year-old son, mused:

> It is just such a short span. That's what I'm realizing, sitting here answering all these questions. I thought it was not worth it at the time. I remember telling friends, "This is supposed to be wonderful, but I am not impressed one bit with pregnancy." But now I hardly remember the answers to the questions you're asking. I had a lot of those problems, but they faded away.

What causes this fading? A sudden awareness of proportions. First, proportions of time: When you hold your newborn child in your arms, a lifetime stretches ahead—a lifetime that will outlast your own. When you look back over your shoulder at pregnancy, you'll miss it if you blink. Second is the proportion of trial to reward: Nine months of suffering is nothing compared to a lifetime of joy. This is the balance in which everyone who has already had a baby is weighing your pregnancy problems. Unfortunately, that balance is still not available to you, because you still don't know what the joy will be.

After all, how can you set your sights on the future when the future is so hard to pull into focus? No matter how many babies you count among your close acquaintances, everything about your coming child is completely unknown—what he or she will look like, act like, *feel* like, and how you'll feel in return. No matter how vivid your imagination, it can produce only the faintest glimmers of what you will experience the first time you hold your baby—or the second, or the fiftieth, or the ten thousandth time. The transforming power of parenthood is simply inaccessible to those who have not yet become parents. About all you can do is listen to those who have been transformed.

Said Diane:

> Your children are the only thing—at least that I've found—that tugs at your heart, that you see yourself in, that makes you laugh one minute and cry the next. I can't believe what a wonderful, emotional thing it is. It's the only thing that makes me break down and weep in happiness. The only thing.

And Bonnie:

> As hard as a pregnancy may be, the moments I gave birth to each of my children were the most beautiful moments of my life. The beauty of your child makes it all worth any pain or discomfort. The joy they bring in the years to come is worth it all. My children have blessed my life with more joy than I could ever have imagined.

And Barbara:

> I feel complete. I mean, my children add a dimension to my life that I can't even put into words—though I wish I could.

And Kate:

> Being a mother is the most fun I've ever had, and I have had a very fun life. No matter how happy I am to see my son go off to sleep at night, I am always thrilled by him all over again when he wakes up the next morning. It's always another day of surprises. I never know what he's going to say or do that will make me laugh or just leave me goggle-eyed in amazement. And I've grown so much. I do things for him that I didn't know I could do. I feel like we're growing up together.

And Kim D.:

> It's so trite to say that it's all well worth it, but once you get that child in your arms, once you see them yawn or smile or grab a toy, you are mesmerized and nothing else matters.
>
> To watch a child develop into a "real" person, with a favorite color and music, et cetera, is the most miraculous thing. My favorite thing to do is sit back and watch my kids figure something out. Whether it's opening a Tupperware container, peeling the paper from a crayon, or playing with a puzzle, there's nothing more exciting than watching those chubby fingers, that determined face, and those little eyes that light up with success. It's better than anything else on earth.

And it is way, way better than being pregnant. Linda Sue, writing again after the birth of her daughter, thinks so, too:

> When I look at my daughter, I fill with such love and pride. She is so perfect and beautiful. It is difficult to grasp that my body housed this perfect little angel, that all the nausea, fatigue, soreness, pain, and the rest of the discomforts were because of her!
>
> Julia Sue came exactly three weeks past my due date. All the discomforts in the world couldn't prepare me for what became an extra month of pregnancy! But when I looked at her for the first time, my heart melted. How can you stay angry at such a little and helpless being? Now that my child was a reality, rather than an abstract *in utero*, I was glad I had endured it.
>
> She is seven weeks old now. Most of the particulars of my troubles and discomforts have faded. I do remember it was horrendous. However, if I were to look at the survey I answered for this book I'm sure I would be saying to myself, "Really? I felt that?" or, "Oh, yeah, now I remember."
>
> As Julia and I become better at breastfeeding (something else of which no one shares the pain and anxieties!) I fall deeper in love. All the discomforts I felt during pregnancy do not negate the fact that my body nourished her, helped her grow and develop. And I continue to do so. It is a wonderful experience. I'm glad I did it—once!

Once, twice, ten times—the wonder will be there for you. So good luck. Joy is coming to you. Be ready to take it.

Appendix

VIEWS ON EXERCISE IN PREGNANCY ARE currently undergoing a good deal of reexamination in the medical community. Whereas pregnant women were once counseled to avoid regular physical activity, within the last twenty-five years that advice has changed, possibly because many women in American society, having discovered the pleasures and benefits of regular exercise, cannot be persuaded to abandon it at a time when their bodies most need care and attention. In 1985, the American College of Obstetricians and Gynecologists (ACOG) released a set of guidelines for exercise in pregnancy. These guidelines involved rather strict limitations, but in 1994, they were revised to allow for more activity as many doctors became convinced that in normal pregnancy the benefits of regular exercise outweigh the risks.

The most obvious and demonstrable benefit is increased maternal fitness. The logical assumption is that this improved fitness has a beneficial effect on other aspects of pregnancy, including self-image, physical symptoms, labor course, and recovery. However, none of these benefits has been conclusively demonstrated.[1]

The subject of exercise in pregnancy thus remains somewhat controversial. Doctors are understandably reluctant to give a universal green light to activity that carries even the potential for risk in pregnancy. However, for the most part, the potential dangers have not been reliably demonstrated.

The many ways in which pregnancy circumvents apparently problematic situations are still not understood. Furthermore, both exercise and pregnancy provoke significant and complex changes in the internal environment; when you combine the two, the interaction becomes deeply complex and the results unpredictable.[2] Factors that influence that interaction include type, duration, and intensity of exercise, the exterior environment (for example, is the room hot or cold?), the fitness level of the woman, and the point in the pregnancy.[3] You should take all of these factors into account, along with the potential risks, when you consider what types and amounts of exercise will be appropriate for you.

Perhaps the most common reason women used to be advised against exercise in pregnancy was the demonstrable fact that exercise diverts blood from the internal organs to the muscles. In earlier years doctors assumed this diversion would be harmful to the fetus, but that assumption has not been borne out by studies of women who exercise in moderation during pregnancy. Evidently there are compensatory mechanisms that protect the fetus from the effects of decreased blood flow.[4]

However, you will probably feel the effects of pregnancy-related changes in your cardiovascular system. Exercise produces predictable responses in the heart and blood vessels, including increases in blood volume, cardiac output, and resting pulse. In a pregnant woman, all these factors are already increased by the pregnancy itself, so if you try to exercise to your nonpregnant levels you may feel more easily overwhelmed by the same amount of effort. At the same time, exercise decreases the squeezing force of the blood vessels, which in normal pregnancy is already considerably reduced. Because this low blood pressure puts a pregnant woman at greater risk for lightheadedness, you should be especially careful about sudden posture changes while exercising (such as quick changes from sitting to standing positions).

The respiratory system of a pregnant woman is under stress and consumes more oxygen than when she is not pregnant. Aerobic exercise, of course, increases oxygen consumption as well. Be aware that the oxygen you take in will be less available to your exercising muscles. The results can include breathlessness and easy exhaustion. If you are accustomed to vigorous exercise, you may feel more comfortable if you reduce your level of aerobic activity to compensate for the respiratory changes of pregnancy.

Exercise elevates body temperature, and doctors once feared that such elevation would place the fetus at risk. However, as in the case of diverted blood flow, evidence indicates that such fears are not justified. The mother's body is already producing extra heat in pregnancy because of the higher basal metabolic rate, but doctors note that the body adapts to this heat in a way that apparently protects or benefits the fetus.[5] Furthermore, research suggests that in physically fit women, exercise does not elevate core temperatures.[6]

Another concern about exercise involves pregnancy's effects on the musculoskeletal system. First of all, a pregnant woman is simply out of balance. Her usual center of gravity is displaced, requiring her to learn new ways of standing and moving. At the same time, hormones produce a general increase of looseness and mobility in the joints, making them less reliable. These effects are to be taken seriously in your choice of exercise, especially in sports requiring balance, strength, swift movement, and rapid changes of direction—for example, tennis, skiing, or gymnastics.[7] (See below for remarks on other sports.) However, it is possible that women who exercise regularly before pregnancy and maintain some version of their exercise regimen throughout pregnancy have fewer musculoskeletal injuries and complaints in pregnancy than women who do not exercise.[8]

In general, beginning exercise before pregnancy and continuing it on a regular basis seems to provide the greatest benefits. The 1994 recommendations of the ACOG[9] state that pregnant women should

- ***pursue mild to moderate exercise on a regular basis (at least three times a week).*** *Intermittent exercise is much less beneficial than regular exercise, especially for women who are sedentary before pregnancy.*

- ***avoid exercising on their backs.*** *This is important because in this position, by the second trimester, the uterus impedes the flow of blood from the lower body back to the heart. Also, pregnant women should avoid standing for long periods, which also impedes blood flow.*

- ***modify activity to compensate for the increased oxygen consumption of pregnancy.*** *A woman should not exercise to the point of exhaustion. Weight-bearing exercise, such as walking or aerobic dance, is fine in most cases, but non-weight-bearing exercise, such as swimming, offers better protection from injury—and an injured woman can't maintain her exercise routine.*

- ***avoid exercise where loss of balance would result in injury, especially to the abdominal area, and anything else that puts the abdominal area at risk for blows and falls.***

- ***increase caloric intake, especially in carbohydrates.*** *Maintaining a pregnancy requires at least 300 extra calories a day, and physical activity only increases that requirement.*

- ***avoid becoming overheated while exercising.*** *Any exercising woman, pregnant or not, should drink water as needed, wear loose, cool clothing, and avoid workouts in a room that feels excessively warm or stuffy.*

- ***remember that the body changes of pregnancy persist for about four to six weeks postpartum.*** *Any pregnancy-related adjustments in an exercise routine should continue for at least one month after delivery.*

Specific activities on which doctors advise caution include contact sports and basketball (because of the potential for abdominal trauma); skiing, ice-skating, gymnastics, horseback riding, and climbing (because of the potential for joint injury or falls); water skiing (which can force water into the genital tract); and scuba diving (which carries a risk for the formation of nitrogen bubbles in the bloodstream). Weight training, generally good for pregnant women, should never involve strain and should not include exercises performed lying on the back.[10]

In certain cases, the risks of exercise may outweigh the benefits. The ACOG guidelines state that exercise is probably not suitable in cases of

- *pregnancy-induced hypertension,*
- *premature rupture of membranes,*
- *preterm labor (in previous or current pregnancy),*
- *incompetent cervix, and*
- *intrauterine growth retardation.*[11]

If any of these circumstances applies to your pregnancy, do not exercise without careful consultation with your physician.

You should also consult your doctor before exercising if you have a preexisting physical condition such as a heart abnormality, hypertension, or a musculoskeletal disorder. Because there is virtually no information available on how these conditions might interact with exercise in pregnancy, your physician will probably advise extreme caution. It is worth noting that research suggests exercise in pregnancy may help to control preexisting or gestational diabetes by inducing a low blood sugar state; however, existing studies on this possibility are limited.[12]

Finally, be aware that much of the existing research on exercise in pregnancy has been conducted with subjects who were reasonably fit before becoming pregnant. Research on women with extremely sedentary lifestyles who begin exercise in pregnancy is almost nonexistent.[13] If you have been habitually very sedentary, do not begin even a moderate exercise program without first checking with your doctor.

Notes

1

Nausea and Vomiting

1. Thomas L. Abell and Caroline A. Riely, "Hyperemesis Gravidarum," *Gastroenterology Clinics of North America* 21, no. 4 (December 1992): 835.
2. M. M. Weigel and R. M. Weigel, "The Association of Reproductive History, Demographic Factors, and Alcohol and Tobacco Consumption with the Risk of Developing Nausea and Vomiting in Early Pregnancy," *American Journal of Epidemiology* 127, no. 3 (March 1988): 563.
3. Cited by Denys V. I. Fairweather, "Nausea and Vomiting in Pregnancy," *American Journal of Obstetrics and Gynecology* 102, no. 1 (September 1, 1968): 160.
4. This remark was quoted in a handout from the Natural Baby Company regarding nausea and vomiting in pregnancy. A free copy of this handout is available from the company at (609) 771-9233.
5. R. Swaminathan, R. K. Chin, T. T. H. Lao, Y. T. Mak, N. S. Panesar, and C. S. Cockram, "Thyroid Function in Hyperemesis Gravidarum," *Acta Endocrinologica* 120 (1989): 155–160.
6. R. K. H. Chin and T. T. H. Lao, "Thyroxine Concentration and Outcome of Hyperemetic Pregnancies," *British Journal of Obstetrics and Gynaecology* 95 (May 1988): 508.
7. P. Johnson, G. Samsioe, and A. Gustafson, "Studies in Cholestasis of Pregnancy, Part I: Clinical Aspects and Liver Function Tests," *Acta Obstetricia et Gynecologica Scandinavica* 54 (1975): 79.
8. A. Järnfelt-Samsioe, G. Samsioe, and G. M. Velinder, "Nausea and Vomiting in Pregnancy—A Contribution to Its Epidemiology," *Gynecologic and Obstetric Investigation* 16 (1983): 221.
9. Järnfelt-Samsioe, Samsioe, and Velinder, 227.
10. R. R. Schade, M. J. Pelekanos, W. N. Tauxe, and D. H. Van Thiel, "Gastric Emptying Time During Pregnancy," abstract, *Gastroenterology* 86 (1984): 1234.
11. M. Mogadam, "Perspective as to Pathogenesis and Management of Hyperemesis in Pregnancy," letter, *American Journal of Gastroenterology* 87, no. 6 (June 1992): 806–808.
12. A. E. Czeizel, I. Dudas, G. Fritz, A. Tescoi, A. Hanck, and G. Kunovits, "The Effect of Periconceptional Multivitamin-mineral Supplementation on Vertigo, Nausea and Vomiting in the First Trimester of Pregnancy," *Archives of Gynecology and Obstetrics* 251, no. 4 (1992): 181–185.
13. G. Samsioe, N. Crona, L. Enk, and A. Järnfelt-Samsioe, "Does Position and Size of Corpus Luteum Have Any Effect on Nausea of Pregnancy?" *Acta Obstetricia et Gynecologica Scandinavica* 65 (1986): 427–429.

14. J. M. Thorp, Jr., W. J. Watson, and V. L. Katz, "Effect of Corpus Luteum Position on Hyperemesis Gravidarum: A Case Report," *Journal of Reproductive Medicine* 36 (October 1991): 761–762.
15. "Does Position and Size of Corpus Luteum Have Any Effect on Nausea and Vomiting of Pregnancy?" Editorial, *Obstetrical and Gynecological Survey* 42, no. 8 (May 1987): 494–495.
16. Vol. 42, no. 8 (May 1987): 495.
17. Fairweather, 160.
18. Fairweather, 136.
19. Mogadam, 807.
20. G. M. Iatrakis, G. G. Sakellaropoulos, A. H. Kourkoubas, and S. E. Kabounia, "Vomiting and Nausea in the First Twelve Weeks of Pregnancy," *Psychotherapy and Psychosomatics* 49, no. 1 (1988): 22–24.
21. This chart is drawn from information in Mary C. Brucker, "Management of Common Minor Discomforts in Pregnancy, Part III: Managing Gastrointestinal Problems in Pregnancy," *Journal of Nurse-Midwifery* 33, no. 2 (March/April 1988): 68–69.
22. Elisabeth Hyde, "Acupressure Therapy for Morning Sickness: A Controlled Clinical Trial," *Journal of Nurse-Midwifery* 34, no. 4 (July/August 1989): 171–178.
23. V. Sahakian, D. Rouse, S. Sipes, N. Rose, and J. Niebyl, "Vitamin B_6 Is Effective Therapy for Nausea and Vomiting of Pregnancy: A Randomized, Double-blind Placebo-controlled Study," *Obstetrics and Gynecology* 78 (July 1991): 33–36.
24. Ione Sims, "Coping with Nausea in Pregnancy," *Mothering* (Winter 1984): 56.
25. W. Fischer-Rasmussen, S. K. Kjaer, C. Dahl, and U. Asping, "Ginger Treatment of Hyperemesis Gravidarum," *European Journal of Obstetrics, Gynecology, and Reproductive Biology* 38 (January 4, 1991): 23.
26. Fairweather, 150.

2

Headache

1. Audrey Uknis and Stephen D. Silberstein, "Review Article: Migraine and Pregnancy," *Headache* 31 (June 1991): 372–374.
2. For example, see K. M. A. Welch, "Migraine: A Biobehavioral Disorder," *Cephalalgia*, Suppl. 4 (1986): 104; and Michael A. Moskowitz, "The Neuorobiology of Vascular Head Pain," *Annals of Neurology* 16 (1984): 157.
3. D. A. Marcus, "Serotonin and Its Role in Headache Pathogenesis and Treatment," *Clinical Journal of Pain* 9, no. 3 (September 1993): 162.
4. J. C. Tinajero, A. Fabbri, D. A. Ciocca, and M. L. Dufau, "Serotonin Secretion from Rat Leydig Cells," *Endocrinology* 133, no. 6 (December 1993): 3026.
5. K. M. A. Welch, "Migraine and Pregnancy," in *Neurological Complications of Pregnancy*, ed. by O. Devinsky, E. Feldmann, and B. Hainline (New York: Raven, 1994): 80.
6. Charles W. Theisler, *Migraine Headache Disease: Diagnostic and Management Strategies* (Gaithersburg, MD: Aspen, 1990): 32.
7. Stephen D. Silberstein and George R. Merriam, "Estrogens, Progestins, and Headache," *Neurology* 41 (1991): 787.

8. L. A. Salamonsen and J. K. Findlay, "Regulation of Endometrial Prostaglandins During the Menstrual Cycle and in Early Pregnancy," *Reproduction, Fertility, and Development* 2, no. 5 (1990): 446.
9. Theisler, 34.
10. Theisler, 147.
11. Marcus, 164.
12. Cited in Theisler, 103.
13. Theisler, 105.
14. Mary Darling, "Exercise and Migraine: A Critical Review," *Journal of Sports Medicine and Physical Fitness* 31, no. 2 (June 1991): 295–296.
15. Theisler, 124.
16. N. Vijayan, "Headband for Migraine Headache Relief," *Headache* 33 (January 1993): 40–41.
17. George Vozar, "Nonpharmacological Treatment of Headache," letter, *Headache* 33 (September 1993): 455.
18. M. Gans, "Treating Migraine by 'Sleep-rationing,'" *Journal of Nervous and Mental Disease* 113 (1951): 405–429.
19. Berkeley: University of California Press, 1985.
20. L. C. Turner, J. F. Rothrock, and C. A. Molgaard, "A Neural Shift Theory of Migraine," *Neuroepidemiology* 12, no. 4 (1993): 249–250.
21. Sacks, 198.

3

Mood Disorders

1. Quoted in Kent Kyger and Warren W. Webb, "Progesterone Levels and Psychological State in Normal Women," *American Journal of Obstetrics and Gynecology* 113, no. 6 (July 15, 1972): 759.
2. Barbara L. Parry and Sarah L. Berga, "Neuroendocrine Correlates of Behavior During the Menstrual Cycle," Chapter 58 in Vol. 3 of *Psychiatry*, ed. by Robert Michels et al. (Philadelphia: Lippincott, 1993): 4.
3. Dyane D. Affonso, Steven Lovett, Steven Paul, Suann Sheptak, Rhoda Nussbaum, Lawrence Newman, and Bruce Johnson, "Dysphoric Distress in Childbearing Women," *Journal of Perinatology* 12, no. 4 (1992): 325–332.
4. W. Wuttke, M. Arnold, D. Becker, O. D. Creutzfeldt, S. Langenstein, S. Poppl, and W. Tirsch, "Changes in the EEG During Menstrual Cycle of Women with and Without Oral Contraceptives," abstract, *Progress in Brain Research* 42 (1975): 322–323; and D. Becker, M. Arnold, O. D. Creutzfeldt, S. Langenstein, and W. Wuttke, "Variations of Performance in Psychological Tests During the Menstrual Cycle in Women with and Without Oral Contraceptives," abstract, *Progress in Brain Research* 42 (1975): 323.
5. Francis J. Kane, Jr., Robert J. Daly, John A. Ewing, and Martin H. Keeler, "Mood and Behavioural Changes with Progestational Agents," *British Journal of Psychiatry* 113 (1967): 265.
6. Kenneth S. Kendler, Nicholas G. Martin, Andrew C. Heath, David Handelsman, and Lindon J. Eaves, "A Twin Study of the Psychiatric Side Effects of Oral Contraceptives," *Journal of Nervous and Mental Disease* 176, no. 3 (1988): 153–160.

7. Ali Jarrahi-Zadeh, F. J. Kane, Jr., R. L. Van de Castle, A. Lachenbruch, and J. A. Ewing, "Emotional and Cognitive Changes in Pregnancy and Early Puerperium," *British Journal of Psychiatry* 115 (1969): 802–803.
8. Cited in Jarrahi-Zadeh, Kane, et al., 803.
9. These examples are from studies cited in Jarrahi-Zadeh, Kane, et al., 803.
10. From a study cited in Kane, Daly, et al., 266.
11. Lorah D. Dorn, Elizabeth J. Susman, and Anne C. Petersen, "Cortisol Reactivity and Anxiety and Depression in Pregnant Adolescents: A Longitudinal Perspective," *Psychoneuroendocrinology* 18, no. 3 (1993): 219–229.
12. Karen A. Matthews and Judith Rodin, "Pregnancy Alters Blood Pressure Response to Psychological and Physical Challenge," *Psychophysiology* 29, no. 2 (1992): 232–240.
13. John A. Pilgrim, Stephen Stansfield, and Michael Marmot, "Low Blood Pressure, Low Mood?" *BMJ* 304 (January 11, 1992): 75.
14. See Paul Gilbert, *Depression: From Psychology to Brain State* (Hillsdale, NJ: Lawrence Erlbaum, 1984): especially chapter 5, "Psycho-neurochemical Approaches."
15. M. I. Assael, J. M. Namboze, G. A. German, and F. J. Bennett, "Psychiatric Disturbances During Pregnancy in a Rural Group of African Women," *Social Science and Medicine* 6 (1972): 388.
16. Lowell F. Bushnell, "First-trimester Depression: A Suggested Treatment," *Obstetrics and Gynecology* 18, no. 3 (September 1961): 282.
17. Bushnell, 281.
18. Affonso, 326.
19. S. Suzuki, L. Dennerstein, K. M. Greenwood, S. M. Armstrong, T. Sano, and E. Satohisa, "Melatonin and Hormonal Changes in Disturbed Sleep During Late Pregnancy," *Journal of Pineal Research* 15 (1993): 192.
20. Barbara L. Parry, Norman E. Rosenthal, Lawrence Tamarkin, and Thomas A. Weir, "Treatment of a Patient with Seasonal Premenstrual Syndrome," *American Journal of Psychiatry* 144, no. 6 (June 1987): 762–765.
21. Yung Sik Chung and Amin N. Daghestani, "Seasonal Affective Disorder: Shedding Light on a Dark Subject," *Postgraduate Medicine* 86, no. 5 (October 1989): 310–311.
22. Parry, Rosenthal, et al., 765.
23. A. Byrne and D. G. Byrne, "The Effect of Exercise on Depression, Anxiety and Other Mood States: A Review," *Journal of Psychosomatic Research* 37, no. 6 (1993): 566.
24. Michael Baumblatt and Frank Winston, "Pyridoxine and the Pill," letter, *Lancet* 1, no. 651 (April 18, 1970): 832–833.
25. Herbert Schamburg, Jerry Kaplan, Anthony Windebank, Nicholas Vick, Stephen Rasmus, David Pleasure, and Mark J. Brown, "Sensory Neuropathy from Pyridoxine Abuse: A New Megavitamin Syndrome," *New England Journal of Medicine* 309, no. 8 (August 25, 1983): 445–448.
26. John H. Greist and James W. Jefferson, *Depression and Its Treatment* (Washington, DC, and London: American Psychiatric Press, 1992): 79.
27. Richard J. Shader, "Question the Experts: 'Does Continuous Use of Fluoxetine During the First Trimester Present a High Risk . . . ?'" *Journal of Clinical Pyschopharmacology* 12, no. 6 (December 1992): 441.

28. Lawrence L. Kerns, "Treatment of Mental Disorders in Pregnancy: A Review of Psychotropic Drug Risks and Benefits," *Journal of Nervous and Mental Disease* 174, no. 11 (November 1, 1986): 655–656.
29. Kerns, 656–657.

4

Fatigue

1. By J. Pritchard, P. MacDonald, and N. Gant (Norwalk, CT: Appleton-Century-Crofts, 1985).
2. Jacqueline Fawcett and Ruth York, "Spouses' Physical and Psychological Symptoms During Pregnancy and the Postpartum," *Nursing Research* 35, no. 3 (May/June 1986): 146.
3. Carol J. Poole, "Fatigue During the First Trimester of Pregnancy," *Journal of Obstetric, Gynecologic, and Neonatal Nursing* 15, no. 5 (September/October 1986): 375.
4. Nedra Reeves, Kathleen Potempa, and Agatha Gallo, "Fatigue in Early Pregnancy: An Exploratory Study," *Journal of Nurse-Midwifery* 36, no. 5 (September/October 1991): 303–309.
5. Reeves, Potempa, and Gallo, 307.
6. Reeves, Potempa, and Gallo, 307.
7. Poole, 375.
8. Poole, 377.
9. Arlene M. Wallace, Diane B. Boyer, Alice Dan, and Karen Holm, "Aerobic Exercise, Maternal Self-esteem, and Physical Discomforts During Pregnancy," *Journal of Nurse-Midwifery* 31, no. 6 (November/December 1986): 255–262.
10. Poole, 377.
11. Michael J. Baumblatt and Frank Winston, "Pyridoxine and the Pill," *Lancet* 1, no. 65 (April 18, 1970): 832–833.
12. Herbert Schamberg, Jerry Kaplan, Anthony Windebank, Nicholas Vick, Stephen Rasmus, David Pleasure, and Mark J. Brown, "Sensory Neuropathy from Pyridoxine Abuse: A New Megavitamin Syndrome," *New England Journal of Medicine* 309, no. 8 (August 25, 1983): 445–448.

5

Sleep Disturbances

1. Marshall D. Lindheimer, William M. Baron, Jacques Durr, and John M. Davison, "Water Homeostasis and Vasopressin Release During Rodent and Human Gestation," *American Journal of Kidney Diseases* 9, no. 4 (April 1987): 270.
2. Avital Fast, Lyn Weiss, Sheilesh Parikh, and Gila Hertz, "Night Backache in Pregnancy: Hypothetical Pathophysiological Mechanisms," *American Journal of Physical Medicine and Rehabilitation* 68, no. 5 (October 1989): 227.
3. Thomas S. Ross, "Night Cramps," *Australian Family Physician* 17, no. 7 (July 1988): 533.
4. J. S. Black, "Night Cramps," letter, *Australian Family Physician* 17, no. 11 (November 1988): 941.

5. McParland and J. Malcolm Pearce, "Restless Legs Syndrome in Pregnancy: Case Reports," *Clinical and Experimental Obstetrics and Gynecology* 1 p 6.
6. P. McParland and Pearce, 6.
7. Fast, Weiss, Parikh, and Hertz, 227–228.
8. I. L. Thomas, J. Nicklin, H. Pollock, and K. Faulkner, "Evaluation of a Maternity Cushion (Ozzlo Pillow) for Backache and Insomnia in Late Pregnancy," *Australian and New Zealand Journal of Obstetrics and Gynecology* 29 (1989): 135.
9. Richard X. Sands, "Backache of Pregnancy: A Method of Treatment," *Obstetrics and Gynecology* 12, no. 6 (December 1958): 670.
10. Ismet Karacan, Wayne Heine, Harman W. Agnew, Jr., Robert L. Williams, Wilse B. Webb, and John J. Ross, "Characteristics of Sleep Patterns During Late Pregnancy and the Postpartum Periods," *American Journal of Obstetrics and Gynecology* 101, no. 5 (July 1, 1968): 584.
11. M. W. Johns, T. J. Gay, J. Masterson, et al., "Relationship Between Sleep Habits, Adrenocortical Activity and Personality," *Psychosomatic Medicine* 33 (November/December 1971): 409–508.
12. O. Petre-Quadens, A. M. De Barsy, J. Devos, and Z. Sfaello, "Sleep in Pregnancy: Evidence of Foetal-sleep Characteristics," *Journal of Neurological Science* 4 (1967): 600–605.
13. S. Suzuki, L. Dennerstein, K. M. Greenwood, S. M. Armstrong, T. Sano, and E. Satohisa, "Melatonin and Hormonal Changes in Disturbed Sleep During Late Pregnancy," *Journal of Pineal Research* 15 (1993): 191–198.

6

Heartburn

1. Todd H. Baron and Joel E. Richter, "Gastroesophageal Reflux Disease in Pregnancy," *Gastroenterology Clinics of North America* 21, no. 4 (December 1992): 781–782.
2. J. M. Marrero, M. Goggin, J. S. de Caestecker, J. M. Pearce, and J. D. Maxwell, "Determinants of Pregnancy Heartburn," *British Journal of Obstetrics and Gynaecology* 99 (September 1992): 731–734.
3. Cited in Marrero, Goggin, et al., 733.
4. Joel E. Richter, "Heartburn, Dysphagia, Odynophagia, and Other Esophageal Symptoms," Chapter 17 in *Gastrointestinal Disease: Pathophysiology/Diagnosis/Management*, ed. by Marvin H. Sleisenger and John S. Fordtran (Philadelphia: Saunders, 1993): 336.
5. Baron and Richter, 786–789.

7

Bell's Palsy

1. Cited in Anand D. Deshpande, "Recurrent Bell's Palsy in Pregnancy," *Journal of Laryngology and Otology* 104 (September 1990): 714.
2. Anne D. Walling, "Bell's Palsy in Pregnancy and the Puerperium," *Journal of Family Practice* 36, no. 5 (1993): 562.

8

Ear, Nose, Throat, and Mouth Problems

1. M. Bende, U. Hallgårde, C. Sjögren, and K. Uvnäs-Moberg, "Nasal Congestion During Pregnancy," *Clinical Otolaryngology* 14, no. 5 (October 1989): 385–387.
2. D. McShane and M. A. Walsh, "Nasal Granuloma Gravidarum," *Journal of Laryngology and Otology* 102, no. 9 (September 1988): 830.
3. Craig S. Derkay, "Eustachian Tube and Nasal Function During Pregnancy: A Prospective Survey," *Otolaryngology–Head and Neck Surgery* 99, no. 6 (December 1988): 564.
4. Derkay, 564.
5. Tom D. Daley, Nii O. Nartey, and George Wysocki, "Pregnancy Tumor: An Analysis," *Oral Surgery, Oral Medicine, Oral Pathology* 72, no. 2 (1991): 196–199.

10

Feet and Legs

1. Gerard J. Kerbleski and James W. Moore, "Management of Pedal Changes Encountered with Pregnancy," *Journal of the American Podiatric Medical Association* 79, no. 7 (July 1989): 340.
2. J. S. Black, "Night Cramps," letter, *Australian Family Physician* 17, no. 11 (November 1988): 941.
3. Kerbleski and Moore, 342–343.
4. R. Alvarez, I. A. F. Stokes, D. E. Asprinio, S. Trevino, and T. Braun, "Dimensional Changes of the Feet in Pregnancy," *Journal of Bone and Joint Surgery* 70–A, no. 2 (February 1988): 271–274.

11

Backache

1. Brian Hainline, "Low-back Pain in Pregnancy," in *Neurological Complications of Pregnancy*, ed. by O. Devinsky, E. Feldmann, and B. Hainline (New York: Raven, 1994): 65.
2. Quoted by Joseph Alcalay and John E. Wolf, Jr., "Pruritic Urticarial Papules and Plaques of Pregnancy: The Enigma and the Confusion," *Journal of the American Academy of Dermatology* 19, no. 6 (December 1988): 1115. The quoted passage is Genesis 3:16.
3. Richard X. Sands, "Backache of Pregnancy: A Method of Treatment," *Obstetrics and Gynecology* 12, no. 6 (December 1958): 670.
4. Cited in Hainline, 66.
5. Avital Fast, Lyn Weiss, Edmond J. Ducommun, Evelyn Medina, and John G. Butler, "Low-back Pain in Pregnancy: Abdominal Muscles, Sit-up Performance, and Back Pain," *Spine* 15, no. 1 (1990): 28–30.
6. Avital Fast, Daniel Shapiro, Edmond J. Ducommun, Lawrence W. Friedmann, Thalia Bouklas, and Yizhar Floman, "Low-back Pain in Pregnancy," *Spine* 12, no. 4 (1987): 370.

7. Hainline, 74.
8. Hainline, 68.
9. Nikolai Bogduk, "The Lumbar Disc and Low Back Pain," *Neurosurgery Clinics of North America* 2, no. 4 (October 1991): 799.
10. Hainline, 70.
11. Sands, 670–676.
12. J. M. Daly, S. Frame, and A. Rapoza, "Sacroiliac Sublaxation: A Common, Treatable Cause of Low-back Pain in Pregnancy," *Family Practice Research Journal* 11, no. 2 (June 1991): 149–159.
13. Hainline, 73.
14. Hainline, 73–74.
15. Arlene M. Wallace, Diane B. Boyer, Alice Dan, and Karen Holm, "Aerobic Exercise, Maternal Self-Esteem, and Physical Discomforts During Pregnancy," *Journal of Nurse-Midwifery* 31, no. 6 (November/December 1986): 260.
16. Fast, Weiss, et al., 30.
17. Hainline, 74–75.
18. All exercises described by Hainline, 75.
19. Cited in Hainline, 74.
20. Cited in Daniel C. Cherkin, "Family Physicians and Chiropractors: What's Best for the Patient?" *Journal of Family Practice* 35, no. 5 (1992): 505.
21. Peter Curtis and Geoffrey Bove, "Family Physicians, Chiropractors, and Back Pain," *Journal of Family Practice* 35, no. 5 (1992): 553.
22. Joseph R. DiPalma and G. John DiGregorio, "Management of Low Back Pain by Analgesics and Adjuvant Drugs," *Mount Sinai Journal of Medicine* 58, no. 2 (March 1991): 101.
23. Cited in Richard Deyo, "Nonsurgical Care of Low Back Pain," *Neurosurgery Clinics of North America* 2, no. 4 (October 1991): 856.
24. H. L. Rosomoff and R. S. Rosomoff, "Comprehensive Multidisciplinary Pain Center Approach to the Treatment of Low Back Pain," *Neurosurgery Clinics of North America* 2, no. 4 (October 1991): 882.
25. H. C. Ostgaard, G. B. J. Andersson, and M. Wennergren, "The Impact of Low Back and Pelvic Pain in Pregnancy on the Pregnancy Outcome," *Acta Obstetricia et Gynecologica Scandinavica* 70, no. 1 (1991): 21.

12

Carpal Tunnel Syndrome

1. J. S. Wand, "Carpal Tunnel Syndrome in Pregnancy and Lactation," *Journal of Hand Surgery* 15, no. 1 (February 1990): 94.
2. John L. Melvin, Carolyn N. Burnett, and Ernest W. Johnson, "Median Nerve Conduction in Pregnancy," *Archives of Physical Medicine and Rehabilitation* 50 (February 1969): 78.
3. Cited in N. Soferman, S. L. Weissman, and M. Haimov, "Acroparesthesias in Pregnancy," *American Journal of Obstetrics and Gynecology* 89, no. 4 (June 15, 1964): 530.
4. Soferman, Weissman, and Haimov, 529.
5. William E. Crisp and Salvatore DeFrancesco, "The Hand Syndrome of Pregnancy," *Obstetrics and Gynecology* 23, no. 3 (March 1964): 436.
6. Crisp and DeFrancesco, 437.

13

Edema

1. Vern L. Katz, Rebecca M. Ryder, Robert C. Cefalo, Stephanie C. Carmichael, and Robert Goolsby, "A Comparison of Bed Rest and Immersion for Treating the Edema of Pregnancy," *Obstetrics and Gynecology* 75, no. 2 (February 1990): 147.
2. Katz, Ryder, et al., 147–151.
3. Katz, Ryder, et al., 150.

14

Bowel Problems

1. Annie S. Anderson, "Dietary Factors in the Aetiology and Treatment of Constipation During Pregnancy," *British Journal of Obstetrics and Gynaecology* 93 (March 1986): 247.
2. N. Levy, E. Lemberg, and M. Sharf, "Bowel Habit in Pregnancy," *Digestion* 4 (1971): 216.
3. Anderson, 247.
4. Anderson, 248.
5. Edmund W. Godding, "Laxatives and the Special Role of Senna," *Pharmacology* 36, Suppl. 1 (1988): 232.
6. Thrift G. Hanks, "Milk as Obstipant," letter, *JAMA* 230, no. 4 (October 28, 1974): 538–539.
7. Arlene Wallace, Diane B. Boyer, Alice Dan, and Karen Holm, "Aerobic Exercise, Maternal Self-esteem, and Physical Discomforts During Pregnancy," *Journal of Nurse-Midwifery* 31, no. 6 (November/December 1986): 259.
8. Linda West, Jeff Warren, and Teresa Cutts, "Diagnosis and Management of Irritable Bowel Syndrome, Constipation, and Diarrhea in Pregnancy," *Gastroenterology Clinics of North America* 21, no. 4 (December 1992): 797.
9. Levy, Lemberg, and Sharf, 220.
10. Godding, 232.
11. Godding, 230.
12. Andrea Jacobs Singer and Lawrence J. Brandt, "Pathophysiology of the Gastrointestinal Tract During Pregnancy," *American Journal of Gastroenterology* 86, no. 12 (1991): 1707.
13. James H. Lewis, Allan B. Weingold, and the Committee on FDA-Related Matters, "The Use of Gastrointestinal Drugs During Pregnancy and Lactation," *American Journal of Gastroenterology* 80, no. 11 (1985): 914.
14. Godding, 231–232.
15. Lewis, Weingold, and the Committee on FDA-Related Matters, 914.
16. Susun Weed, *Wise Woman Herbal for the Childbearing Year* (Woodstock, NY: Ash Tree, 1986).
17. Levy, Lemberg, and Sharf, 216.
18. Levy, Lemberg, and Sharf, 221.
19. West, Warren, and Cutts, 794.
20. Levy, Lemberg, and Sharf, 222.

21. West, Warren, and Cutts, 795.
22. West, Warren, and Cutts, 797–798.
23. West, Warren, and Cutts, 795.

15

Skin Problems

1. Cited in John V. Dacus, "Pruritus in Pregnancy," *Clinical Obstetrics and Gynecology* 33, no. 4 (December 1990): 738.
2. Cited in Ann G. Martin and Susana Leal-Khouri, "Physiologic Skin Changes Associated with Pregnancy," *International Journal of Dermatology* 31, no. 6 (June 1992): 375.
3. D. Kemmett and M. J. Tidman, "The Influence of the Menstrual Cycle and Pregnancy on Atopic Dermatitis," *British Journal of Dermatology* 125, no. 1 (1991): 60.
4. Kemmett and Tidman, 60.
5. The first published use of this name was by T. J. Lawley, K. C. Hertz, T. R. Wade, A. B. Ackerman, and S. I. Katz, "Pruritic Urticarial Papules and Plaques of Pregnancy," *JAMA* 241 (1979): 1696–1699. Cited in Joseph Alcalay and John E. Wolf, "Pruritic Urticarial Papules and Plaques of Pregnancy: The Enigma and the Confusion," *Journal of the American Academy of Dermatology* 19, no. 6 (December 1988): 1115.
6. Alcalay and Wolf, 1115.
7. The first published use of this name was by R. C. Holmes and M. M. Black, "The Specific Dermatoses of Pregnancy," *Journal of the American Academy of Dermatology* 8 (1983): 405–412. Cited in Alcalay and Wolf, 1115.
8. Lisa M. Cohen, Eleanor L. Capeless, Paul A. Krusinski, and Mary E. Maloney, "Pruritic Urticarial Papules and Plaques of Pregnancy and Its Relationship to Maternal-fetal Weight Gain and Twin Pregnancy," *Archives of Dermatology* 125 (November 1989): 1534–1536.
9. Robert Weiss and Peter Hull, "Familial Occurrence of Pruritic Urticarial Papules and Plaques of Pregnancy," *Journal of the American Academy of Dermatology* 26 (1992): 715–717.
10. K. B. Yancey, R. Hall, and T. J. Lawley, "Pruritic Urticarial Papules and Plaques of Pregnancy," *Journal of the American Academy of Dermatology* 10 (1984): 475–476.
11. Jeffrey K. Shornick, "Herpes Gestationis," *Journal of the American Academy of Dermatology* 17, no. 4 (October 1987): 540.
12. Cited in Shornick, 541.
13. Cited in Shornick, 552.
14. Cited in Dacus, 741.
15. John C. Murray, "Pregnancy and the Skin," *Dermatologic Clinics* 8, no. 2 (April 1990): 332.
16. Dacus, 743.
17. Martin and Leal-Khouri, 376.
18. Martin and Leal-Khouri, 376.
19. Diane J. Madlon-Kay, "Striae Gravidarum: Folklore and Fact," *Archives of Family Medicine* 2, no. 2 (May 1993): 507.
20. Cited in Madlon-Kay, 507.

21. Madlon-Kay, 510, 511.
22. Tim Parmley and Timothy J. O'Brien, "Skin Changes During Pregnancy," *Clinical Obstetrics and Gynecology* 33, no. 4 (December 1990): 715.

Appendix

1. James F. Clapp III, Roxanne Rokey, Judith L. Treadway, Marshall W. Carpenter, Raul M. Artal, and Carole Warrnes, "Exercise in Pregnancy," *Medicine and Science in Sports and Exercise* 24, no. 6, Supplement (1992): s296.
2. Clapp, Rokey, et al., s294.
3. Clapp, Rokey, et al., s295.
4. Betsy Schick-Boshetto and Nancy C. Rose, "Exercise and Pregnancy," *Obstetrical and Gynecological Survey* 47, no. 1 (1991): 10.
5. "ACOG Issues Recommendations on Exercise During Pregnancy and the Postpartum Period," *American Family Physician* 49, no. 5 (April 1994): 1258–1259.
6. Cited in Schick-Boshetto and Rose, 11.
7. Raul Artal, "Exercise and Pregnancy," *Clinics in Sports Medicine* 11, no. 2 (April 1992): 365.
8. Clapp, Rokey, et al., s296.
9. "ACOG Issues Recommendations," 1258–1259.
10. Schick-Boshetto and Rose, 12.
11. "ACOG Issues Recommendations," 1259.
12. Clapp, Rokey, et al., s297.
13. Clapp, Rokey, et. Al., s298.

Bibliography

Abell, T. L. "Nausea and Vomiting of Pregnancy and the Electrogastrogram: Old Disease, New Technology." Editorial; comment. *American Journal of Gastroenterology* 87 (June 1992): 689–691.

Abell, T. L., and C. A. Riely. "Hyperemesis Gravidarum." *Gastroenterology Clinics of North America* 21 (December 1992): 835–849.

"ACOG Issues Recommendations on Exercise During Pregnancy and the Post-partum Period." *American Family Physician* 49, no. 5 (April 1994): 1258–1259.

Affonso, Dyanne D., Steven Lovett, Steven Paul, Suann Sheptak, Rhoda Nussbaum, Lawrence Newman, and Bruce Johnson. "Dysphoric Distress in Childbearing Women." *Journal of Perinatology* 12, no. 4 (December 1992): 325–332.

Akiskal, Hagop Souren. "The Clinical Management of Affective Disorders." Chapter 61 in Vol. 1 of *Psychiatry*, ed. by Robert Michels et al. Philadelphia: Lippincott, 1993.

Alcalay, Joseph, and John E. Wolf, Jr. "Pruritic Urticarial Papules and Plaques of Pregnancy: The Enigma and the Confusion." *Journal of the American Academy of Dermatology* 19, no. 6 (December 1988): 1115–1116.

Alvarez, R., I. A. F. Stokes, D. E. Asprinio, S. Trevino, and T. Braun. "Dimensional Changes of the Feet in Pregnancy." *Journal of Bone and Joint Surgery* 70–A, no. 2 (February 1988): 271–274.

Anderson, Annie S. "Dietary factors in the Aetiology and Treatment of Constipation During Pregnancy." *British Journal of Obstetrics and Gynecology* 93 (March 1986): 245–249.

Archer, David F. "Physiology of Prolactin." *Clinical Obstetrics and Gynecology* 23, no. 2 (June 1980): 325–335.

Artal, Raul. "Exercise and Pregnancy." *Clinics in Sports Medicine* 11, no. 2 (April 1992): 363–377.

Assael, M. I., J. M. Namboze, G. A. German, and F. J. Bennett. "Psychiatric Disturbances During Pregnancy in a Rural Group of African Women." *Social Science and Medicine* 6 (1972): 387–395.

Bahna, Sami L., and Douglas C. Heiner. *Allergies to Milk*. New York: Grune and Stratton, 1980.

Barclay, B. A. "Experience with Enteral Nutrition in the Treatment of Hyperemesis Gravidarum." *Nutrition in Clinical Practice* 5 (August 1990): 153–155.

Baron, Todd H., and Joel E. Richter. "Gastroesophageal Reflux Disease in Pregnancy." *Gastroenterology Clinics of North America* 21, no. 4 (December 1992): 777–791.

Baumblatt, Michael, and Frank Winston. "Pyridoxine and the Pill." Letter. *Lancet* 1, no. 651 (April 18, 1970): 832–833.

Beary, John F., and Herbert Benson. "A Simple Psychophysiologic Technique Which Elicits the Hypometabolic Changes of the Relaxation Response." *Psychosomatic Medicine* 36, no. 2 (March–April 1974): 115–120.

Beaton, J. G. "Nausea of Pregnancy: A 'Natural' Remedy.' *Postgraduate Medicine* 74 (November 1983): 50.

Bebbington, Paul E. "Psychosocial Etiology of Schizophrenia and Affective Disorders." Chapter 63 in Vol. 1 of *Psychiatry*, ed. by Robert Michels et al. Philadelphia: Lippincott, 1993.

Becker, D., P. M. Arnold, O. D. Creutzfeldt, S. Langenstein, and W. Wuttke. "Variations of Performance in Psychological Tests During the Menstrual Cycle in Women with and Without Oral Contraceptives." Abstract in *Progress in Brain Research* 42 (1975): 323.

Bende, M., U. Hallgårde, C. Sjögren, and K. Uvnäs-Moberg. "Nasal Congestion During Pregnancy." *Clinical Otolaryngology* 14, no. 5 (October 1989): 385–387.

Bennett, A. "Prostaglandins: Their Release, Biological Effects and Relationships to Pain and Inflammation." *Cephalalgia* 6, Suppl. 4 (1986): 17–20.

Bergan, John J. "Varicose Veins: Chronic Venous Insufficiency." Chapter 42 in *Vascular Surgery: A Comprehensive Review*, ed. by Wesley S. Moore. 4th ed. Philadelphia: Saunders, 1993.

Berlin, Richard M. "Sleepwalking Disorder During Pregnancy: A Case Report." *Sleep* 11, no. 3 (June 1988): 298–300.

Bernstein, A. L. "Vitamin B_6 in Clinical Neurology." *Annals of the New York Academy of Sciences* 585 (1990): 250–260.

Black, J. S. "Night Cramps." Letter. *Australian Family Physician* 17, no. 11 (November 1988): 941.

Bogduk, Nikolai. "The Lumbar Disc and Low Back Pain." *Neurosurgery Clinics of North America* 2, no. 4 (October 1991): 791–806.

Boyce, R. A. "Enteral Nutrition in Hyperemesis Gravidarum: A New Development." *Journal of the American Dietetic Association* 92 (June 1992): 733–736.

Braverman, Lewis E., and Robert D. Utiger. "Introduction to Thyrotoxicosis." Chapter 30 in Werner and Ingbar's *The Thyroid: A Fundamental and Clinical Text*, ed. by Lewis E. Braverman and Robert D. Utiger. 6th ed. Philadelphia: Lippincott, 1991.

Brewerton, T. D., and M. S. George. "A Study of the Seasonal Variation of Migraine." *Headache* 30, no. 8 (July 1990): 511–513.

Brucker, Mary C. "Management of Common Minor Discomforts in Pregnancy. Part III: Managing Gastrointestinal Problems in Pregnancy." *Journal of Nurse-Midwifery* 33 (March–April 1992): 67–73.

Burd, Laurence I., Melvin Dorin, Vimala Philipose, and James A. Lemons. "The Relationship of Mammary Temperature to Parturition in Human Subjects." *American Journal of Obstetrics and Gynecology* 128, no. 3 (June 1, 1977): 272–278.

Bushnell, Lowell F. "First–trimester Depression: A Suggested Treatment." *Obstetrics and Gynecology* 18, no. 3 (September 1961): 281–282.

Byrne, A., and D. G. Byrne. "The Effect of Exercise on Depression, Anxiety, and Other Mood States: A Review." *Journal of Psychosomatic Research* 37, no. 6 (1993): 565–574.

Charbonneau, Marc, Tommaso Falcone, Manuel G. Cosio, and Robert D. Levy. "Obstructive Sleep Apnea During Pregnancy: Therapy and Implications for Fetal Health." *American Review of Respiratory Disease* 144, no. 2 (August 1991): 461–463.

Cherkin, Daniel C. "Family Physicians and Chiropractors: What's Best for the Patient?" *Journal of Family Practice* 35, no. 5 (1992): 505–506.

Chertok, L., M. L. Mondzain, and M. Bonnaud. "Vomiting and the Wish to Have a Child." *Psychosomatic Medicine* 25 (1963): 13–18.

Chin, R. K. "Hyperemesis Gravidarum and Fetal Growth Retardation." Letter. *American Journal of Obstetrics and Gynaecology* 162 (May 1990): 1349.

Chin, R. K. H., and Lao, T. T. H. "Thyroxine Concentration and Outcome of Hyperemetic Pregnancies." *British Journal of Obstetrics and Gynecology* 95 (May 1988): 507–509.

Chung, Yung Sik, and Amin N. Daghestani. "Seasonal Affective Disorder: Shedding Light on a Dark Subject." *Postgraduate Medicine* 86, no. 5 (October 1989): 309–314.

Clapp, James F.,III, Roxanne Rokey, Judith L. Treadway, Marshall W. Carpenter, Raul M. Artal, and Carole Warrnes. "Exercise in Pregnancy." *Medicine and Science in Sports and Exercise* 24, no. 6, supplement (1992): s294–s300.

Cohen, Lisa M., Eleanor L. Capeless, Paul A. Krusinski, and Mary E. Maloney. "Pruritic Urticarial Papules and Plaques of Pregnancy and Its Relationship to Maternal–fetal Weight Gain and Twin Pregnancy." *Archives of Dermatology* 125 (November 1989): 1534–1536.

Cohen, Sidney. "The Sluggish Gallbladder of Pregnancy." *New England Journal of Medicine* 302 (Feb. 14, 1980): 397–399.

Cox, John L. "Psychiatric Morbidity and Pregnancy: A Controlled Study of 263 Semi–rural Ugandan Women." *British Journal of Psychiatry* 134 (1979): 401–405.

Crisp, William, and Salvatore DeFrancesco. "The Hand Syndrome of Pregnancy." *Obstetrics and Gynecology* 23, no. 3 (March 1964): 433–437.

Curtis, Peter, and Geoffrey Bove. "Family Physicians, Chiropractors, and Back Pain." *Journal of Family Practice* 35, no. 5 (1992): 551–555.

Czeizel, A. E., I. Dudas, G. Fritz, A. Tescoi, A. Hanck, and G. Kunovits. "The Effect of Periconceptional Multivitamin–mineral Supplementation on Vertigo, Nausea, and Vomiting in the First Trimester of Pregnancy." *Archives of Gynecology and Obstetrics* 251 (1992): 181–185.

Dacus, John V. "Pruritus in Pregnancy." *Clinical Obstetrics and Gynecology* 33, no. 4 (December 1990): 738–745.

Daley, Tom D., Nii O. Nartey, and George P. Wysocki. "Pregnancy Tumor: An Analysis." *Oral Surgery, Oral Medicine, Oral Pathology* 72, no. 2 (August 1991): 196–199.

Daly, J. M., P. S. Frame, and P. A. Rapoza. "Sacroiliac Sublaxation: A Common, Treatable Cause of Low-back Pain in Pregnancy." *Family Practice Research Journal* 11, no. 2 (June 1991): 149–159.

Darling, Mary. "Exercise and Migraine: A Critical Review." *Journal of Sports Medicine and Physical Fitness* 31, no. 2 (June 1991): 294–302.

Depue, R. H., L. Bernstein, R. K. Ross, H. L. Judd, and B. E. Henderson. "Hyperemesis Gravidarum in Relation to Estradiol Levels, Pregnancy Outcome, and Other Maternal Factors: A Serioepidemiologic Study." *American Journal of Obstetrics and Gynecology* 156 (May 1987): 1137–1141.

Derkay, Craig S. "Eustachian Tube and Nasal Function During Pregnancy: A Prospective Study." *Otolaryngology–Head and Neck Surgery* 99, no. 6 (December 1988): 558–566.

Deshpande, Anand. "Recurrent Bell's Palsy in Pregnancy." *Journal of Laryngology and Otology* 104 (September 1990): 713–714.

Dexter, J. D. "The Relationship Between Stage III, IV, and REM Sleep and Arousals with Migraine." *Headache* 19 (1979): 364–369.

Deyo, Richard A. "Nonsurgical Care of Low Back Pain." *Neurosurgery Clinics of North America* 2, no. 4 (October 1991): 851–862.

Diamant, N. E. "Physiology of the Esophagus." Chapter 16 in *Gastrointestinal Disease: Pathophysiology/Diagnosis/Management*, ed. by Marvin H. Sleisenger and John S. Fordtran. Philadelphia: Saunders, 1993.

Diamond, Seymour. "Strategies for Migraine Management." *Cleveland Clinical Journal of Medicine* 58, no. 3 (May–June 1991): 257–261.

DiPalma, Joseph R., and G. John DiGregorio. "Management of Low Back Pain by Analgesics and Adjuvant Drugs." *Mount Sinai Journal of Medicine* 58, no. 2 (March 1991): 101–105.

"Does Position and Size of Corpus Luteum Have Any Effect on Nausea and Vomiting of Pregnancy?" Editorial. *Obstetrical and Gynecological Survey* 42 (May 1987): 494–495.

Dorn, Lorah D., Elizabeth J. Susman, and Anne C. Petersen. "Cortisol Reactivity and Anxiety and Depression in Pregnant Adolescents: A Longitudinal Perspective." *Psychoneuroendocrinology* 18, no. 3 (1993): 219–239.

Dunner, David L. "Affective Disorders: Clinical Features." Chapter 59 in Vol. 1 of *Psychiatry*, ed. by Robert Michels et al. Philadelphia: Lippincott, 1993.

Ekman–Ordeberg, Gunvar, Stig Salgeback, and Gunnar Ordeberg. "Carpal Tunnel Syndrome in Pregnancy: A Prospective Study." *Acta Obstetricia et Gynecologica Scandinavica* 66 (1987): 233–235.

Ella, Josephine, Ira R. Katz, and George M. Simpson. Introduction. "Teratogenicity of Psychotherapeutic Medications." *Psychopharmacology Bulletin* 23, no. 4 (1987): 531–532.

Elliott, S. A., A. J. Rugg, J. P. Watson, and D. I. Brough. "Mood Changes During Pregnancy and After the Birth of a Child." *British Journal of Clinical Psychology* 22 (1983): 295–308.

el–Mallakh, R. S., N. R. Liebowitz, and M. S. Hale. "Hyperemesis Gravidarum as Conversion Disorder." *Journal of Nervous and Mental Disease* 178 (October 1990): 655–659.

Everson, Gregory T. "Gastrointestinal Motility in Pregnancy." *Gastroenterology Clinics of North America* 21, no. 4 (December 1992): 751–775.

Fairweather, D. V. I. "Nausea and Vomiting in Pregnancy."*American Journal of Obstetrics and Gynecology* (September 1, 1968): 135–175.

Fast, Avital, Daniel Shapiro, Edmond J. Ducommun, Lawrence W. Friedmann, Thalia Bouklas, and Yizhar Floman. "Low-back Pain in Pregnancy." *Spine* 12, no. 4 (1987): 368–371.

Fast, Avital, Lyn Weiss, Edmond J. Ducommun, Evelyn Medina, and John G. Butler. "Low-back Pain in Pregnancy: Abdominal Muscles, Sit-up Performance, and Back Pain." *Spine* 15, no. 1 (1990): 28–30.

Fast, Avital, Lyn Weiss, Sheilesh Parikh, and Gila Hertz. "Night Backache in Pregnancy: Hypothetical Pathophysiological Mechanisms." *American Journal of Physical Medicine and Rehabilitation* 68, no. 5 (October 1989): 227–229.

Fawcett, Jacqueline, and Ruth York. "Spouses' Physical and Psychological Symptoms During Pregnancy and the Postpartum." *Nursing Research* 35, no. 3 (May/June 1986): 144–148.

Feinsilver, Steven H., and Gila Hertz. "Respiration During Sleep in Pregnancy." *Clinics in Chest Medicine* 13, no. 4 (December 1992): 637–644.

Fischer-Rasmussen, W., S. K. Kjaer, C. Dahl, and U. Asping. "Ginger Treatment of Hyperemesis Gravidarum." *European Journal of Obstetrics, Gynecology, and Reproductive Biology* 38 (January 4, 1991): 19–24.

Friedan, Betty. *The Feminine Mystique*. New York: Norton, 1963.

Gallery, Eileen D. M. "Volume Homeostasis in Normal and Hypertensive Human Pregnancy." *Seminars in Nephrology* 4, no. 3 (September 1984): 221–229.

Gans, M. "Treating Migraine by 'Sleep-rationing.' *Journal of Nervous and Mental Disease* 113 (1951): 405–429.

Gilbert, Paul. *Depression: From Psychology to Brain State*. Hillsdale NJ: Lawrence Erlbaum, 1984.

Gillin, J. Christian. "Sleep and Dreams." Chapter 60 in Vol. 3 of *Psychiatry*, ed. by Robert Michels et al. Philadelphia: Lippincott, 1993.

Godding, Edmund W. "Laxatives and the Special Role of Senna." *Pharmacology* 36, Supplement 1 (1988): 230–236.

Godsey, R. K., and R. B. Newman. "Hyperemesis Gravidarum: A Comparison of Single and Multiple Admissions." *Journal of Reproductive Medicine* 35 (April 1991): 287–290.

Goodwin, T. M., M. Montoro, and J. H. Mestman. "Transient Hyperthyroidism and Hyperemesis Gravidarum: Clinical Aspects." *American Journal of Obstetrics and Gynecology* 167 (September 1992): 648–652.

Greist, John H., and James W. Jefferson. *Depression and Its Treatment*. Washington, DC: American Psychiatric Press, 1992.

Gross, S., C. Librach, and A. Cecutti. "Maternal Weight Loss Associated with Hyperemesis Gravidarum: A Predictor of Fetal Outcome." *American Journal of Obstetrics and Gynecology* 160 (April 1989): 906–909.

Gudholdt, I. S., B. G. Trolle, and L. E. Hvidman. "Iron Supplementation During Pregnancy." *Acta Obstetricia et Gynecologica Scandinavica* 70, no. 1 (1991): 9–12.

Hainline, Brian. "Low-back Pain in Pregnancy." In *Neurological Complications of Pregnancy*. Ed. by O. Devinsky, E. Feldmann, and B. Hainline. New York: Raven, 1994.

Hanks, Thrift G. "Milk as Obstipant." Letter. 230, no. 4 (October 28, 1974): 538–539.

Harvey, W. A., and M. J. Sherfey. "Vomiting in Pregnancy: A Psychiatric Study." *Psychosomatic Medicine* 16 (1954): 1–9.

Hertz, Gila, Avital Fast, Steven H. Feinsilver, Claude L. Albertario, Harold Schulman, and Alan M. Fein. "Sleep in Normal Late Pregnancy." *Sleep* 15, no. 3 (June 1992): 246–251.

Hilliard, P. A. "Coping with Morning Sickness." *Parents'* 65 (August 1990).

Holmes, R. C., and M. M. Black. "The Specific Dermatoses of Pregnancy." *Journal of the American Academy of Dermatology* 8 (1983): 405–412.

Holroyd, Kenneth A., and Donald B. Penzien. "Pharmacological Versus Non–-pharmacological Prophylaxis of Recurrent Migraine Headache: A Meta-analytic Review of Clinical Trials." *Pain* 42 (1990): 1–13.

Hyde, E. "Acupressure Therapy for Morning Sickness: A Controlled Clinical Trial." *Journal of Nurse-Midwifery* 34 (July/August 1989): 171–178.

Iatrakis, G. M., G. G. Sakellaropoulos, A. H. Kourkoubas, and S. E. Kabounia. "Vomiting and Nausea in the First Twelve Weeks of Pregnancy." *Psychotherapy and Psychosomatics* 49 (1988): 22–24.

Järnfelt-Samsioe, A. "Nausea and Vomiting in Pregnancy: A Review." *Obstetrical and Gynecological Survey* 41 (1987): 422–427.

Järnfelt-Samsioe, A., B. Erikkson, K. H. Lessner, and G. Samsioe. "Gallbladder Disease Related to Use of Oral Contraceptives and Nausea in Pregnancy." *Southern Medical Journal* 78 (September 1985): 1040–1043.

Järnfelt-Samsioe, A., G. Samsioe, and G. M. Velinder. "Nausea and Vomiting in Pregnancy: A Contribution to Its Epidemiology." *Gynecologic and Obstetric Investigation* 16 (1983): 221–229.

Jarrahi-Zadeh, Ali, F. J. Kane, Jr., R. L. Van de Castle, P. A. Lachenbruch, and J. A. Ewing. "Emotional and Cognitive Changes in Pregnancy and the Early Puerperium." *British Journal of Psychiatry* 115 (1969): 797–805.

Jick, S. S., and J. M. Garrison. "Discontinuation of Bendectin." *American Journal of Public Health* 78 (March 1988): 322–323.

Johns, M. W., T. J. Gay, J. P. Masterson, et al. "Relationship Between Sleep Habits, Adrenocortical Activity and Personality." *Psychosomatic Medicine* 33 (November–December 1971): 499–508.

Johnson, P., G. Samsioe, and A. Gustafson. "Studies in Cholestasis of Pregnancy. Part I: Clinical Aspects and Liver Function Tests." *Acta Obstetricia et Gynecologica Scandinavica* 54 (1975): 77–84.

Kahrilas, Peter J., and Walter J. Hogan. "Gastrointestinal Reflux Disease." Chapter 19 in *Gastrointestinal Disease: Pathophysiology/Diagnosis/Management*, ed. by Marvin H. Sleisenger and John S. Fordtran. Philadelphia: Saunders, 1993.

Kane, Francis J., Jr., Robert J. Daly, John A. Ewing, and Martin H. Keeler. "Mood and Behavioural Changes with Progestational Agents." *British Journal of Psychiatry* 113 (1967): 265–268.

Karacan, Ismet, Wayne Heine, Harman W. Agnew, Jr., Robert L. Williams, Wilse B. Webb, and John J. Ross. "Characteristics of Sleep Patterns During Late Pregnancy and the Postpartum Period." *American Journal of Obstetrics and Gynecology* 101, no. 5 (July 1, 1968): 579–586.

Katon, W. J., R. K. Ries, J. A. Bokan, and Arthur Kleinman. "Hyperemesis Gravidarum: A Biopsychosocial Perspective." *International Journal of Psychiatry in Medicine* 10 (1980–81): 151–162.

Katz, Vern L., Tammy Jenkins, Leigh Haley, and Watson A. Bowes, Jr. "Catecholamine Levels in Pregnant Physicians and Nurses: A Pilot Study of Stress and Pregnancy." *Obstetrics and Gynecology* 77, no. 3 (March 1991): 338–342.

Katz, Vern L., Lynda Rozas, Rebecca Ryder, and Robert C. Cefalo. "Effect of Daily Immersion on the Edema of Pregnancy." *American Journal of Perinatology* 9, no. 4 (July 1992): 225–227.

Katz, Vern L., Rebecca M. Ryder, Robert C. Cefalo, Stephanie C. Carmichael, and Robert Goolsby. "A Comparison of Bed Rest and Immersion for Treating the Edema of Pregnancy." *Obstetrics and Gynecology* 75, no. 2 (February 1990): 147–151.

Kemmett, D., and M. J. Tidman. "The Influence of the Menstrual Cycle and Pregnancy on Atopic Dermatitis." *British Journal of Dermatology* 125, no. 1 (1991): 59–61.

Kendler, Kenneth S., Nicholas G. Martin, Andrew C. Heath, David Handelsman, and Lindon J. Eaves. "A Twin Study of the Psychiatric Side Effects of Oral Contraceptives." *Journal of Nervous and Mental Disease* 176, no. 3 (1988): 153–160.

Kennedy, R. L., J. Darne, R. Davies, and A. Price. "Thyrotoxicosis and Hyperemesis Gravidarum Associated with a Serum Activity Which Stimulates Human Thyroid Cells in Vitro." *Clinical Endocrinology* 36 (January 1992): 83–89.

Kerbleski, Gerard J., and James W. Moore. "Management of Pedal Changes Encountered with Pregnancy." *Journal of the American Podiatric Medical Association* 79, no. 7 (July 1989): 340–344.

Kerns, Lawrence L. "Treatment of Mental Disorders in Pregnancy: A Review of Psychotropic Drug Risks and Benefits." *Journal of Nervous and Mental Disease* 174, no. 11 (Nov. 1, 1986): 652–659.

Kerr, M. G., D. B. Scott, and Eric Samuel. "Studies of the Inferior Vena Cava in Late Pregnancy." *British Medical Journal* 1 (1964): 532–533.

"Key Witness Against Morning Sickness Drug Faces Scientific Fraud Charges." *JAMA* 263 (March 16, 1990): 1468–1469.

Kuller, J. M. "Effects on the Fetus and Newborn of Medications Commonly Used During Pregnancy." *Journal of Perinatal and Neonatal Nursing* 3 (April 1990): 73–87.

Kutner, S. Jerome, and Willard L. Brown. "History of Depression as a Risk Factor for Depression with Oral Contraceptives and Discontinuance." *Journal of Nervous and Mental Disease* 155, no. 3 (1972): 163–169.

Kyger, Kent, and Warren W. Webb. "Progesterone Levels and Psychological State in Normal Women." *American Journal of Obstetrics and Gynecology* 113, no. 6 (July 15, 1972): 759–762.

LaBan, Myron M. "Analysis of Nocturnal Back Pain in Pregnancy." Letter. *American Journal of Physical Medicine and Rehabilitation* 69, no. 2 (April 1990): 108.

LaBan, Myron M., Sherry L. Viola, Anothony F. Femminineo, and Ronald S. Taylor. "Restless Legs Syndrome Associated with Diminished Cardiopulmonary Compliance and Lumbar Spinal Stenosis—a Motor Concomitant of 'Vesper's Curse.'" *Archives of Physical Medicine and Rehabilitation* 71 (May 1990): 384–388.

Lao, T. T., R. K. H. Chin, Y. T. Mak, and N. S. Panesar. "Plasma Zinc Concentration and Thyroid Function in Hyperemetic Pregnancies." *Acta Obstetricia et Gynecologica Scandinavica* 67 (1988): 599–604.

Laros, Russell K., Jr. "Hypertensive Disorders During Pregnancy." Chapter 26 in *Obstetrics and Gynecology*, ed. by J. Robert Wilson, Elsie Reid Carrington, et al. St Louis: Mosby Year Book, 1991.

Lawson, M., F. Kern, Jr., and G. T. Everson. "Gastrointestinal Transit Time in Human Pregnancy: Prolongation in the Second and Third Trimesters Followed by Postpartum Normalization." *Gastroenterology* 89 (1985): 996–999.

Levy, N., E. Lemberg, and M. Sharf. "Bowel Habit in Pregnancy." *Digestion* 4 (1971): 216–222.

Lewis, D. O. "Hypnoanalgesia for Chronic Pain: The Response to Multiple Inductions at One Session and to Separate Single Inductions." *Journal of the Royal Society of Medicine* 85 (October 1992): 620–624.

Lewis, James H., Allan B. Weingold, and the Committee on FDA-Related Matters, American College of Gastroenterology. "The Use of Gastrointestinal Drugs During Pregnancy and Lactation." *American Journal of Gastroenterology* 80, no. 11 (1985): 912–923.

Lindheimer, Marshall D., William M. Baron, Jacques Durr, and John M. Davison. "Water Homeostasis and Vasopressin Release During Rodent and Human Gestation." *American Journal of Kidney Diseases* 9, no. 4 (April 1987): 270–275.

Loretz, Christopher A., and Howard A. Bern. "Prolactin and Osmoregulation in Vertebrates: An Update." *Neuroendocrinology* 35 (1982): 292–304.

Lowe, T. W., and F. G. Cunningham. "Pregnancy and Thyroid Disease." *Clinical Obstetrics and Gynecology* 34 (March 1991): 72–81.

Lowinger, Paul. Letter. "Prostaglandins and Organic Affective Syndrome." *American Journal of Psychiatry* 146, no. 12 (December 1989): 1647.

MacMullen, Nancy, Laura A. Dulski, and Bonnie Pappalardo. "Antepartum Vulnerability: Stress, Coping, and a Patient Support Group." *Journal of Perinatal and Neonatal Nursing* 6, no. 3 (December 1992): 15–25.

McParland, P., and J. Malcolm Pearce. "Restless Legs Syndrome in Pregnancy: Case Reports." *Clinical and Experimental Obstetrics and Gynecology* 17, no. 1 (1990): 5–6.

McShane, D. P., and M. A. Walsh. "Nasal Granuloma Gravidarum." *Journal of Laryngology and Otology* 102, no. 9 (September 1988): 828–830.

Madlon-Kay, Diane J. "Striae Gravidarum: Folklore and Fact." *Archives of Family Medicine* 2, no. 2 (May 1993): 507–511.

Majerus, P. J., S. B. Guze, W. B. Delong, and E. Robins. "Psychologic Factors and Psychiatric Disease in Hyperemesis Gravidarum: A Follow-up Study of 69 Vomiters and 66 Controls." *International Journal of Psychiatry in Medicine* 10 (November 1960): 421–428.

"Mal de Mère: Simple Remedies Best for Morning Sickness." *FDA Consumer* 22 (November 1988): 26–29.

Malmgren, Rigmor. "The Central Serotoninergic System." *Cephalalgia* 10 (August 1990): 199–204.

Mandel, Steven. "Hemiplegic Migraine in Pregnancy." *Headache* 28, no. 6 (1988): 414–416.

Marcus, D. A. "Serotonin and Its Role in Headache Pathogenesis and Treatment." *Clinical Journal of Pain* 9, no. 3 (September 1993): 159–167.

Marrero, J. M., P. M. Goggin, J. S. de Caestecker, J. M. Pearce, and J. D. Maxwell. "Determinants of Pregnancy Heartburn." *British Journal of Obstetrics and Gynaecology* 99 (September 1992): 731–734.

Martin, Ann G., and Susana Leal-Khouri. "Physiologic Skin Changes Associated with Pregnancy." *International Journal of Dermatology* 31, no. 6 (June 1992): 375–378.

Martin, Mary C., Robert N. Taylor, and John L. Kitzmiller. "The Endocrinology of Pregnancy." Chapter 13 in *Basic and Clinical Endocrinology*, ed. by Francis N. Greenspan and John D. Baxter. 4th ed. Norwalk, CT: Appleton & Lange, 1994.

Massey, E. Wayne. "Migraine During Pregnancy." *Obstetrical and Gynecological Survey* 32, no. 11 (1977): 693–696.

Masson, G. M., F. Anthony, and E. Chau. "Serum Chorionic Gonadoptropin (hCG), Schwangerschaftsprotein 1 (SP1), Progesterone and Oestradiol Levels in Patients with Nausea and Vomiting in Early Pregnancy." *British Journal of Obstetrics and Gynecology* 92 (March 1985): 211–215.

Matthews, Karen A., and Judith Rodin. "Pregnancy Alters Blood Pressure Response to Psychological and Physical Challenge." *Psychophysiology* 29, no. 2 (March 1992): 232–240.

Melvin, John L., Carolyn N. Burnett, and Ernest W. Johnson. "Median Nerve Conduction in Pregnancy." *Archives of Physical Medicine and Rehabilitation* 50 (February 1969): 75–80.

Mogadam, M. "Perspective as to Pathogenesis and Management of Hyperemesis in Pregnancy." *American Journal of Gastroenterology* 87 (June 1992): 806–808.

Moskowitz, Michael A. "The Neurobiology of Vascular Head Pain." *Annals of Neurology* 16 (1994): 157–168.

Murray, John C. "Pregnancy and the Skin." *Dermatologic Clinics* 8, no. 2 (April 1990): 327–334.

O'Hara, Michael W. "Social Support, Life Events, and Depression During Pregnancy and the Puerperium." *Archives of General Psychiatry* 43 (June 1986): 569–573.

Osofsky, Joy D., and Howard J. Osofsky. "Pregnancy and New Parenthood: Issues Related to Adjustment and Parental Bonding." Chapter 82 in Vol. 6 of *Gynecology and Obstetrics*, ed. by John J. Sciarra. Philadelphia: Lippincott, 1993.

Ostgaard, H. C., G. B. J. Andersson, and K. Karlsson. "Prevalence of Back Pain in Pregnancy." *Spine* 16, no. 5 (1991): 549–552.

Ostgaard, H. C., G. B. J. Andersson, and M. Wennergren. "The Impact of Low Back and Pelvic Pain in Pregnancy on the Pregnancy Outcome." *Acta Obstetricia et Gynecologica Scandinavica* 70, no. 1(1991): 21–24.

Owman, C., and J. E. Hardebo. "Multiple Transmitter Amines and Peptides in Cerebrovascular Nerves: Possible Links in Migraine Pathophysiology." *Cephalalgia*, Supplement 4 (1986): 49–62.

Palmer, R. L. "A Psychosomatic Study of Vomiting in Early Pregnancy." *Journal of Psychosomatic Research* 17 (1973): 303–308.

Papalos, Demitri, and Papalos, Janice. *Overcoming Depression*. Revised edition. New York: HarperCollins, 1992.

Parmley, Tim, and Timothy J. O'Brien. "Skin Changes During Pregnancy." *Clinical Obstetrics and Gynecology* 33, no. 4 (December 1990): 713–717.

Parry, Barbara L., and Sarah L. Berga. "Neuroendocrine Correlates of Behavior During the Menstrual Cycle." Chapter 58 in Vol. 3 of *Psychiatry*, ed. by Robert Michels et al. Philadelphia: Lippincott, 1993.

Parry, Barbara L., Norman E. Rosenthal, Lawrence Tamarkin, and Thomas A. Weir. "Treatment of a Patient with Seasonal Premenstrual Syndrome." *American Journal of Psychiatry* 144, no. 6 (June 1987): 762–765.

Pastuszak, A., B. Schick–Boschetto., C. Zuber., et al. "Pregnancy Outcome Following First–trimester Exposure to Fluoxetine (Prozac)." *JAMA* 269, no. 17 (May 5, 1993): 2246–2248.

Patton, P. E., and R. L. Stouffer. "Current Understanding of the Corpus Luteum in Women and Nonhuman Primates." *Clinical Obstetrics and Gynecology* 34 (March 1991): 127–139.

Petre–Quadens, O., A. M. De Barsy, J. Devos, and Z. Sfaello. "Sleep in Pregnancy: Evidence of Foetal–sleep Characteristics." *Journal of Neurological Science* 4 (1967): 600–605.

Phillips, Carolyn A. "Vulnerability in Family Systems: Application to Antepartum." *Journal of Perinatal and Neonatal Nursing* 6, no. 3 (December 1992): 26–36.

Pilgrim, John A., Stephen Stansfield, and Michael Marmot. "Low Blood Pressure, Low Mood?" *BMJ* 304 (January 11, 1992): 75–78.

Poole, Carol J. "Fatigue During the First Trimester of Pregnancy." *Journal of Obstetric, Gynecologic, and Neonatal Nursing* 15, no. 5 (September/October 1986): 375–379.

Potter, J. M., and P. J. Nestel. "The Hyperlipidemia of Pregnancy in Normal and Complicated Pregnancies." *American Journal of Obstetrics and Gynecology* 133 (1979): 165–170.

Preskorn, Sheldon H., Carroll W. Hughes, and Steven J. Bupp. "Neurobiological Etiology of Schizophrenic and Affective Disorders." Chapter 64 in Vol. 1 of *Psychiatry*, ed. by Robert Michels et al. Philadelphia: Lippincott, 1993.

Reeves, Nedra, Kathleen Potempa, and Agatha Gallo. "Fatigue in Pregnancy: An Exploratory Study." *Journal of Nurse-Midwifery* 36, no. 5 (September/October 1991): 303–309.

Reik, Louis, Jr. "Headaches in Pregnancy." *Seminars in Neurology* 8, no. 3 (September 1988): 187–192.

Reyniak, J. Victor. "Endocrine Physiology of the Breast." *Journal of Reproductive Medicine* 22, no. 6 (June 1979): 303–309.

Richter, Joel E. "Heartburn, Dysphagia, Odynophagia, and Other Esophageal Symptoms." Chapter 17 in *Gastrointestinal Disease: Pathophysiology/Diagnosis/Management*, ed. by Marvin H. Sleisenger and John S. Fordtran. Philadelphia: Saunders, 1993.

Riezzo, G., et al. "Gastric Myoelectrical Activity in the First Trimester of Pregnancy: A Cutaneous Electrogastrograph Study." *American Journal of Gastroenterology* 87 (June 1992): 702–707.

Robinson, J. E., and R. V. Short. "Changes in Breast Sensitivity at Puberty, During the Menstrual Cycle, and at Parturition." *British Medical Journal* 1 (1977): 1188–1191.

Romrell, Lynn J., and Kirby I. Bland. "Anatomy of the Breast, Axilla, Chest Wall, and Related Metastic Sites." Chapter 2 in *The Breast: Comprehensive Management of Benign and Malignant Disease*, ed. by Kirby I. Bland and Edward M. Copeland III. Philadelphia: Saunders, 1991.

Rosén, L., J. Östergren, B. Fagrell, and E. Stranden. "Mechanisms for Edema Formation in Normal Pregnancy and Preeclampsia Evaluated by Skin Capillary Dynamics." *International Journal of Microcirculation Clinical and Experimental* 9 (1990): 257–266.

Rosenfeld, Jo Ann. "Pregnant Women in the Health Care Professions." *Journal of the American Medical Women's Association* 44, no. 4 (July/August 1989): 119–122.

Rosomoff, H. L., and R. S. Rosomoff. "Comprehensive Multidisciplinary Pain Center Approach to the Treatment of Low Back Pain." *Neuorsurgery Clinics of North America* 2, no. 4 (October 1991): 877–890.

Ross, Thomas S. "Night Cramps." *Australian Family Physician* 17, no. 7 (July 1988): 533.

Rothman, Richard H., and Frederick A. Simone, eds. *The Spine*. 3d ed. Philadelphia: Saunders, 1992.

Sacks, Michael H. "Introduction to the Neuroses." Chapter 31 in Vol. 1 of *Psychiatry*, ed. by Robert Michels et al. Philadelphia: Lippincott, 1993.

Sacks, Oliver. *Migraine: Understanding a Common Disorder*. Berkeley: University of California Press, 1985.

Sahakian, V., D. Rouse, S. Sipes, N. Rose, and J. Niebyl. "Vitamin B_6 Is Effective Therapy for Nausea and Vomiting of Pregnancy: A Randomized, Double-blind Placebo-controlled Study." *Obstetrics and Gynecology* 78 (July 1991): 33–36.

Salamonsen, L. A., and J. K. Findlay. "Regulation of Endometrial Prostaglandins During the Menstrual Cycle and in Early Pregnancy." *Reproduction, Fertility, and Development* 2, no. 5 (1990): 443–457.

Sambrook, M., J. C. Bamber, H. Minasian, and C. R. Hill. "Ultrasonic Doppler Study of the Hormonal Response of Blood Flow in the Normal Human Breast." *Ultrasound in Medicine and Biology* 13, no. 3 (March 1987): 121–129.

Samsioe, G., N. Crona, L. Enk, and A. Järnfelt-Samsioe. "Does Position and Size of Corpus Luteum Have Any Effect on Nausea of Pregnancy?" *Acta Obstetricia et Gynecologica Scandinavica* 65 (1986): 427–428.

Sands, Richard X. "Backache of Pregnancy: A Method of Treatment." *Obstetrics and Gynecology* 12, no. 6 (December 1958): 670–676.

Schade, R. R., M. J. Pelekanos, W. N. Tauxe, and D. H. Van Thiel. "Gastric Emptying Time During Pregnancy." Abstract. *Gastroenterology* 86 (1984): 1234.

Schamburg, Herbert, Jerry Kaplan, Anthony Windebank, Nicholas Vick, Stephen Rasmus, David Pleasure, and Mark J. Brown. "Sensory Neuropathy from Pyridoxine Abuse: A New Megavitamin Syndrome." *New England Journal of Medicine* 309, no. 8 (August 25, 1983): 445–448.

Schick-Boshetto, Betsy, and Nancy C. Rose. "Exercise in Pregnancy." *Obstetrical and Gynecological Survey* 47, no. 1 (1991): 10–13.

Schwartz, Mark Stephen, and Associates. *Biofeedback: A Practitioner's Guide.* New York: Guilford, 1987.

Schweiger, Martin S. "Sleep Disturbance in Pregnancy: A Subjective Survey." *American Journal of Obstetrics and Gynecology* 114, no. 7 (December 1, 1972): 879–882.

Shader, Richard I. "Question the Experts: 'A Patient of Mine Missed a Period While Taking Fluoxetine. . . .'" *Journal of Clinical Psychopharmacology* 12, no. 3 (June 1992): 213.

—. "Question the Experts: 'Does Continuous Use of Fluoxetine During the First Trimester of Pregnancy Present a High Risk?'" *Journal of Clinical Psychopharmacology* 12, no. 6 (December 1992): 441.

Shi, C. Z., and L. Z. Zhuang. "Norepinephrine Regulates Human Chorionic Gonadotropin Production by First Trimester Trophoblast in Vitro." *Placenta* 14, no. 6 (November–December 1993): 683–693.

Shornick, Jeffrey K. "Herpes Gestationis." *Journal of the American Academy of Dermatology* 17, no. 4 (October 1987): 539–556.

Shulman, Adrian, Menahem S. Shapiro, Charles Bahary, and Louis Shenkman. "Abnormal Thyroid Function in Hyperemesis Gravidarum." *Acta Obstetrica et Gynecologica Scandinavica* 68 (1989): 533–536.

Silberstein, Stephen D., and George R. Merriam. "Estrogens, Progestins, and Headache." *Neurology* 41 (June 1991): 786–793.

Sims, Ione. "Coping with Nausea in Pregnancy." *Mothering* (Winter 1984): 55–57.

Singer, Andrea Jacobs, and Lawrence J. Brandt. "Pathophysiology of the Gastrointestinal Tract During Pregnancy." *American Journal of Gastroenterology* 86, no. 12 (1991): 1695–1712.

Skinner, David B., James L. A. Roth, Benjamin H. Sullivan, Jr., George N. Stein, and Mark Levine. "Reflux Esophagitis." Chapter 54 in Vol. 2 of *Backus Gastroenterology*, ed. by J. Edward Berk et al. 4th ed. Philadelphia: Saunders, 1985.

Sleisenger, Marvin H., and John S. Fordtran, eds. *Gastrointestinal Disease: Pathophysiology/Diagnosis/Management.* Philadelphia: Saunders, 1993.

Snyder, Scott. "Unusual Case of Sleep Terror in a Pregnant Patient." Letter. *American Journal of Psychiatry* 143, no. 3 (March 1986): 391.

Soferman, N., S. L. Weissman, and M. Haimov. "Acroparesthesias in Pregnancy." *American Journal of Obstetrics and Gynecology* (June 15, 1964): 528–531.

Sovak, M., M. Kunzel, R. A. Sternbach, and D. J. Dalessio. "Mechanism of the Biofeedback Therapy of Migraine: Volitional Manipulation of the Psychophysiological Background." *Headache* 21, no. 3 (May 1981): 89–92.

Suzuki, S., L. Dennerstein, K. M. Greenwood, S. M. Armstrong, T. Sano, and E. Satohisa. "Melatonin and Hormonal Changes in Disturbed Sleep During Late Pregnancy." *Journal of Pineal Research* 15 (1993): 191–198.

Swaminathan, R., R. K. Chin, T. T. H. Lao, Y. T. Mak, N. S. Panesar, and C. S. Cockram. "Thyroid Function in Hyperemesis Gravidarum." *Acta Endocrinologica* 120 (1989): 155–160.

Telischi, Fred F., and Mark May. "Facial Paralysis of Pregnancy Attributable to an Arteriovenous Steal Syndrome." *American Journal of Otology* 13, no. 4 (July 1992): 375–378.

Thambypillai, V., and K. Staehr–Johansen. "Policies on Iron in Denmark." *Haematologia* 23, no. 3 (1990): 145–149.

Theisler, Charles W. *Migraine Headache Disease: Diagnostic and Management Strategies.* Gaithersburg, MD: Aspen, 1990.

Thomas, I. L., J. Nicklin, H. Pollock, and K. Faulkner. "Evaluation of a Maternity Cushion (Ozzlo Pillow) for Backache and Insomnia in Late Pregnancy." *Australian and New Zealand Journal of Obstetrics and Gynecology* 29, no. 2 (May 1989): 133–138.

Thomson, J. A., R. Wilson, C. Gray, A. C. Glen, and D. Mack. "Hyperemesis Gravidarum and Thyrotoxicosis--A Diagnostic and Therapeutic Problem." *Scottish Medical Journal* 34 (June 1989): 472–473.

Thorp, J. M., Jr., W. J. Watson, and V. L. Katz. "Effect of Corpus Luteum Position on Hyperemesis Gravidarum: A Case Report." *Journal of Reproductive Medicine* 36 (October 1991): 761–762.

Tinajero, J. C., A. Fabbri, D. A. Ciocca, and M. L. Dufau. "Serotonin Secretion from Rat Leydig Cells." *Endocrinology* 133, no. 6 (December 1993): 3026–3029.

Tobin, Sidney M. "Carpal Tunnel Syndrome in Pregnancy." *American Journal of Obstetrics and Gynecology* (February 15, 1967): 493–498.

Torsiglieri, Arthur J., Jr., Lawrence W. C. Tom, William M. Keane, and Joseph P. Atkins, Jr. "Otolaryngologic Manifestations of Pregnancy." *Otolaryngology–Head and Neck Surgery* 102, no. 3 (March 1990): 293–297.

Tur, Ethel, Anat Tamir, and Richard H. Guy. "Cutaneous Blood Flow in Gestational Hypertension and Normal Pregnancy." *Journal of Investigative Dermatology* 99, no. 3 (September 1992): 310–314.

Turner, L. C., J. F. Rothrock, and C. A. Molgaard. "A Neural Shift Theory of Migraine." *Neuroepidemiology* 12, no. 4 (1993): 249–250.

Uddenberg, N., A. Nilsson, and P. E. Almgren. "Nausea in Pregnancy: Psychological and Psychosomatic Aspects." *Journal of Psychosomatic Research* 15 (1971): 269–276.

Uknis, Audrey, and Stephen D. Silberstein. "Review Article: Migraine and Pregnancy." *Headache* 31 (June 1991): 372–374.

van Lier, D., B. Manteuffel, C. Dilorio, and M. Stalcup. "Nausea and Fatigue During Early Pregnancy." *Birth* 20, no. 4 (December 1993): 193–197.

Vijayan, N. "Headband for Migraine Headache Relief." *Headache* 33 (January 1993): 40–41.

Vorherr, Helmuth. "Hormonal and Biochemical Changes of Pituitary and Breast During Pregnancy." *Seminars in Perinatology* 3, no. 3 (July 1979): 193–198.

Vozar, George. "Nonpharmacological Treatment of Headache." Letter. *Headache* 33 (Sept. 1993): 455.

Wallace, Arlene, Diane B. Boyer, Alice Dan, and Karen Holm. "Aerobic Exercise, Maternal Self–esteem, and Physical Discomforts During Pregnancy." *Journal of Nurse–Midwifery* 31, no. 6 (November/December 1986): 255–262.

Walling, Anne D. "Bell's Palsy in Pregnancy and the Puerperium." *Journal of Family Practice* 36, no. 5 (1993): 559–563.

Wand, J. S. "Carpal Tunnel Syndrome in Pregnancy and Lactation." *Journal of Hand Surgery* 15, no. 1 (February 1990): 93–95.

Watson, J. P., S. A. Elliott, A. J. Rugg, and D. I. Brough. "Psychiatric Disorder in Pregnancy and the First Postnatal Year." *British Journal of Psychiatry* 144 (1984): 453–462.

Watts, Nelson B., and Joseph H. Keffer. *Practical Endocrinology*. 4th ed. Philadelphia: Lea and Febiger, 1989.

Weed, Susun. *Wise Woman Herbal for the Childbearing Year*. Woodstock, NY: Ash Tree, 1986.

Weigel, M. M., and R. M. Weigel. "The Association of Reproductive History, Demographic Factors, and Alcohol and Tobacco Consumption with the Risk of Developing Nausea and Vomiting in Early Pregnancy." *American Journal of Epidemiology* 127, no. 3 (March 1988): 562–570.

Weiss, Robert, and Peter Hull. "Familial Occurrence of Pruritic Urticarial Papules and Plaques of Pregnancy." *Journal of the American Academy of Dermatology* 26, no. 5, part I (May 1992): 715–717.

Welch, K. M. A. "Migraine: A Biobehavioral Disorder." *Cephalalgia*, Supplement 4 (1986): 103–110.

—. "Migraine and Pregnancy." In *Neurological Complications of Pregnancy*, ed. by O. Devinsky, E. Feldmann, and B. Hainline. New York: Raven, 1994.

West, Linda, Jeff Warren, and Teresa Cutts. "Diagnosis and Management of Irritable Bowel Syndrome, Constipation, and Diarrhea in Pregnancy." *Gastroenterology Clinics of North America* 21, no. 4 (December 1992): 793–802.

Wright, Phillip E., II. "Carpal Tunnel and Ulnar Tunnel Syndromes and Stenosing Tenosynovitis." Chapter 76 in *Campbell's Operative Orthopaedics*, ed. by A. H. Crenshaw. 8th ed. St. Louis: Mosby Year Book, 1992.

Wuttke, W., P. M. Arnold, D. Becker, O. D. Creutzfeldt, S. Langenstein, S. Pöppl, and W. Tirsch. "Changes in the EEG During Menstrual Cycle of Women with and Without Oral Contraceptives." Abstract. *Progress in Brain Research* 42 (1975): 322–323.

Yancey, K. B., R. P. Hall, and T. J. Lawley. "Pruritic Urticarial Papules and Plaques of Pregnancy." *Journal of the American Academy of Dermatology* 10 (1984): 473–480.

Zierler, S., and K. J. Rothman. "Congenital Heart Disease in Relation to Maternal Use of Bendectin and Other Drugs in Early Pregnancy." *New England Journal of Medicine* 313 (August 8, 1985): 347–352.

Zuckerman, Barry, Hortensia Amaro, Howard Bauchner, and Howard Cabral. "Depressive Symptoms During Pregnancy: Relationship to Poor Health Behaviors." *American Journal of Obstetrics and Gynecology* 160, no. 5 (May 1989): 1107–1111.

Index